MILLIONS OF PEOPLE SUFFER FROM AN EATING DISORDER

"I believed absolutely that I would get everything I wanted if I could be thin. And I developed rituals to make sure I would get there. But the more pounds I lost, the more elaborate the rituals . . . everything began to revolve around food."

"I thought, why not purge? As long as I was still losing weight, I didn't care. Except, everywhere I went, people stared and whispered to each other as I passed. So I thought, well, maybe I've gone a little too far. There was just one problem. I couldn't stop."

"We let our daughter know we were there for her, but we would not watch her kill herself. So we walked into her apartment without knocking. My God, she just dissolved. Right in the middle of the floor, surrounded by all these boxes of junk food . . . I was staggered. My beautiful daughter on the floor, shaking and crying."

From patients, doctors, therapists, and families, these are the words of real people who share their stories as they address the pressing questions: What is anorexia? What is bulimia? How do you fight these debilitating disorders? This guide provides the answers that will help you take the first steps back to health and hope.

THIS BOOK CAN HELP . . .

DYING TO BE THIN

IRA M. SACKER M.D., is an internationally known specialist in the field of eating disorders. In addition to his private practice, he is the Founder/Director of HEED Foundation Inc., a nationally recognized non-profit foundation dedicated to the prevention, education, and treatment of all eating disorders. He is the Director of Adolescent and Young Adult Medicine at the Brookdale University Hospital and Medical Center in New York and has been honored by an appointment to the National Panel on Eating Disorders. Recent appearances on television have included *20/20*, *48 Hours*, the *Today* show, *Good Morning America*, Oprah Winfrey's *Oxygen Network*, all local and national news networks; national and international news; as well as magazines including *People*, *Cosmopolitan*, *Allure*, *Glamour*, *Life* and *Seventeen*. He has published groundbreaking papers on anorexia nervosa, bulimia, and compulsive overeating for medical journals. He has helped develop a new tool for the treatment called Photo and Video-Therapy.

Ira M. Sacker M.D.
Founder/Director of HEED
Helping to End Eating Disorders
10 Sullivan Drive
Jericho, New York 11753
516-822-0324

Director of Eating Disorders
Brookdale University Hospital and
    Medical Center
580 Rockaway Parkway
Brooklyn, New York 11212
718-240-6451

Web site: www.eatingdis.com
E-mail: sackermd@Aol.com

MARC A. ZIMMER, PH.D., holds a Doctorate in Psychology and is a Diplomate in Clinical Social Work. He is the Director of the Biofeedback and Psychotherapy Center in Valley Stream and Brooklyn, NY. There he has specialized in the treatment of eating disorders and stress-related problems for the past twenty years. Dr. Zimmer has developed the integration of biofeedback therapy into a treatment protocol for eating disorders. The author of numerous articles published in professional and educational journals, he has served as both consultant and lecturer to various organizations and is a member of the Benefit Committee of the American Anorexia and Bulimia Association.

Marc A. Zimmer, Ph.D.
Biofeedback and Psychotherapy
    Development, Inc.
5 Sunrise Plaza—Suite #202
Valley Stream, NY 11580
516-825-5005

Brooklyn Location
Biofeedback and Psychotherapy
    Development, Inc.
9229 Flatlands Avenue—2nd Floor
Brooklyn, NY 11236
718-204-0660

DYING TO BE THIN

UNDERSTANDING AND DEFEATING
ANOREXIA NERVOSA AND BULIMIA—A
PRACTICAL, LIFESAVING GUIDE

IRA M. SACKER, M.D.
AND
MARC A. ZIMMER, PH.D.

WARNER BOOKS

A Time Warner Company

WARNER BOOKS EDITION

Copyright © 1987 by Ira M. Sacker, M.D. and Marc A. Zimmer, Ph.D.
Introduction copyright © 1987 by Karola, Inc.
"How Every Teacher Can Help" copyright © 1987 by Roberta Richin, M.A.

Warner Books, Inc., 1271 Avenue of the Americas, New York, NY 10020
Visit our Web site at www.twbookmark.com
For information on Time Warner Trade Publishing's online publishing program, visit www.ipublish.com

 A Time Warner Company

Printed in the United States of Americas
First Printing: August 1987
Reissued: June 2001
20 19 18 17 16 15 14 13 12

Library of Congress Cataloging in Publication Data
Sacker, Ira M.
  Dying to be thin.

  Bibliography
  Includes index.
  1. Anorexia nervosa.   2. Bulimia.   3. Anorexia
nervosa—Case studies.   4. Bulimia—Case studies.
I. Zimmer, Marc A.   II. Title.   [DNLM: 1. Anorexia
Nervosa—popular works.   2. Bulimia—Popular works.
WM 175 S121d]
RC552.A5S23   1987   616.85'2   87-10590
ISBN   0-446-38417-8 (pbk.)

Book design by Giorgetta Bell McRee
Cover design by Martha Sedgwick
Cover photo by Tony Stone/Clarissa Teahy

ATTENTION: SCHOOLS AND CORPORATIONS
WARNER books are available at quantity discounts with bulk purchase for educational, business, or sales promotional use. For information, please write to:
SPECIAL SALES DEPARTMENT, WARNER BOOKS, 1271 AVENUE OF THE AMERICAS, NEW YORK, NY 10020

For Marianne and Hillary, with love.

Acknowledgments

We are grateful to so many people who have given their time, energy, talent, and love to this book. Our families were with us every step of the way, and so we both thank Marianne, Scott, Tara, Harvey and Lottie, Jack and Stella, and Hillary. In addition, there were our patients and their families, who worked so hard to give us the insights and perspective that make this book as much theirs as it is ours.

The same is true for our dear friends and colleagues, Patti and Stephen Englander, Neville Golden, M.D., Jack and Stella, Marvin Surkin, Ph.D., Keith Sedlacek, M.D., Shirley Winston, Ph.D., Barbara Silverman, and Stephen Bronster. They each contributed their concerns, their insights, and most of all—their commitment to the book.

We owe a special debt of gratitude to Dr. Ruth Westheimer, who devoted precious time and thought to this entire project.

Margery Schwartz, our managing editor, and Lillian Rodberg, our copyeditor, worked tirelessly to give this book shape.

And finally, we thank Roberta A. Richin, without whom this book could not have been possible.

Contents

A NOTE TO YOU, THE READER

In a very real sense, this book was written by our patients and those who care about them: parents, teachers, friends. To help you distinguish our comments from their original words, we have printed the text in two kinds of type.

When you see this kind of type, the text consists of our comments.

When you see this kind of type, the text consists of original quotes taken from interviews with patients and others who have directly experienced eating disorders as victims or caring observers.

Preface

Someone you know may literally be dying to be thin. As many as 15 percent of the men and women, boys and girls, who are diagnosed as having anorexia nervosa will die from that disorder this year. An astonishing one in every five college-age women is engaging in some form of bulimic behavior (binging and purging), and the statistics on college-age men continue to climb. No longer a problem limited to a small number of middle and upper-middle class white teenage girls, anorexia and bulimia are insidious and dangerous disorders that can take hold of your life—and even take your life.

Anorexia and bulimia are frightening for all sorts of reasons. These disorders cause painful, long-term health problems, and all sorts of difficulties in relationships. If the symptoms were easy to see, the hazards might be less dramatic. But the symptoms can be very hard to detect, because the person with the eating disorder does such a thorough job of keeping the food and eating behavior a secret.

That is why this book is about secrets. The private world of the anorexic and bulimic is filled with dangerous secrets. Secrets about anger. Guilt. Power. Sexuality. Fear. Growing up.

Self-hatred and self-doubt. People who develop anorexia nervosa or bulimia behaviors work hard and often desperately to keep their behavior secret, even from family whom they live with or see every day.

Concealing intense feelings and self-destructive eating habits can take an extraordinary amount of strength and resourcefulness, so you might think that it would be difficult for a person to keep such a secret for long—especially if that person is someone you care about, whom you might even see every day at home or at work. That's why it is important to establish right from the start that people who suffer from anorexia nervosa or bulimia can successfully hide even the most extreme eating behavior from their parents, spouse, teachers, and friends—even from their doctors.

This person, who could be your child, your student, your friend, or even yourself, can seem to be doing just fine on the outside while suffering immeasurably on the inside. Over the years, virtually hundreds of families, couples, teenagers, parents, women, educators, and doctors have asked us for help in their struggle to see past those outside appearances, to answer the same basic questions:

- What is anorexia?
- What is bulimia?
- What can we do to help?

In each individual case, we developed plans designed to help that particular person find his or her answers. However, the rapid spread of anorexia nervosa and bulimia demands that we all share our insights, and our concerns, in an effort to prevent, identify, and help overcome these eating disorders, because anorexia nervosa and bulimia can take away life itself, claiming more and more people every year.

With the alarming and continuing increase in identified cases of bulimia and anorexia nervosa, we realized that we could reach out to more people more effectively if we developed a book that could accomplish one basic task: to answer the questions that people ask most often about anorexia nervosa and bulimia.

Keeping that goal in mind, we have included a selection of personal histories, fact, and sources so that you can find the information you want easily, in the order you choose. You will learn where to go for support groups, if you are interested in that kind of help, or how to find individual therapy, medical care, guest speakers for school, and training courses to learn more about specific topics.

Some of this information is included in special sections organized by subject. Even more such facts and issues emerge in personal case histories told here by people who have been through great pain, at great cost. These patients and their families decided that it would be valuable for you if they could unmask their secrets so that you could finally understand how some people could become anorexic or bulimic, and how they have worked to recover.

Naturally, all names have been changed to protect the privacy of the people involved. Exceptions to that rule have been made only when the person involved is a public figure—a star of film or television, a model, or a young man or woman who has captured our hearts in athletic competition or dance.

Whether the person you read about is a household word, or a private person whose life may be very much like your own, there is a single, common purpose that holds all of these people together: the shared interest in making sure that you have an opportunity to get some answers to your special questions. Like what causes eating disorders, and how can they be prevented?

All of the answers offered here have been shown to be effective, and all of the cases covered are real. One important thing for you to keep in mind, though, is that *every single person suffering from anorexia nervosa or bulimia is unique*. Treatment that works for one person or family may or may not work for another. That's why we have included a wide variety of individual situations and possible solutions.

No matter how well we might cover a problem, we know that you may have special questions of your own that we do not answer specifically. So you can ask us directly! Just write to us, at the address listed in the Resources section. We welcome your questions, your comments—your feelings.

Ira M. Sacker, M.D.
Marc A. Zimmer, Ph.D.

Introduction
by Dr. Ruth Westheimer

Ever since people started to equate success and beauty with being thin, more and more plans have been developed to help people lose weight, and keep it off.

Some of those plans are very healthy, because they include a balanced emphasis on diet and exercise and mental health. But other diets and weight-loss strategies are not so balanced or healthy. In fact, thousands of young people and adults have become chronically ill and have even died struggling with problems related to food, feelings, and weight loss.

What are some of these diet strategies that can cause so much damage? Starving, bingeing, and purging. Anorexia nervosa is the disorder that involves self-starvation. Bulimia involves bingeing and then purging all the food eaten in the binge. Anorexia nervosa causes people to lose life-threatening amounts of weight because they deny themselves the pleasure of eating, even when they are so hungry that they are in pain. Bulimia may cause people to eat many thousands of calories of food in one sitting, and then purge that food in different ways that can cause terrible health problems and can even lead to death.

Each of these two disorders is very dangerous. There are

times when one person can have symptoms of both difficulties, and may experience numerous and painful complications. Very often, individuals and families struggling with such problems suffer in silence and confusion, wondering what is wrong with them. And it is not just women and young girls who develop these eating disorders! There are men and boys, as well, who develop these same problems, because they too are trying to cope with eating and feelings and weight.

Through all their struggles to cope, anorexic and bulimic people often feel bad about themselves, and wonder if there are others who have similar difficulties. I have found that people tend to feel very bad or ashamed when they think they are the only ones who feel a certain way, or do a certain thing. This is particularly true of people who have anorexia or bulimia.

So many of these young people and adults will use all sorts of elaborate ways to try to hide their illness from people who might not understand. It is very important to know that anorexic and bulimic people do not hide their behavior and their struggle just to be sneaky. They hide because they are often confused, worried, and even ashamed of certain things they do with their own food and hunger and feelings. If they cannot understand it themselves, they often feel it is impossible to tell anyone else, because the other person may ask questions that the bulimic or anorexic person cannot answer.

It is also true that people who are anorexic or bulimic often keep their self-starvation, bingeing, or purging a secret because they do not really know that they have a real and serious disorder that will only get worse if they do not get help. The main problem with keeping such a secret is that anorexia and bulimia only get worse when they are hidden. The more the anorexic or bulimic person pretends that everything is okay, the more the disorder can take over their lives.

The tragedy is that many people struggling to cope with these terrible disorders die, or develop many other chronic and painful physical problems, before anyone else discovers the real disorder.

Sometimes it is very difficult to believe that one little strategy to lose weight or eat big meals without gaining anything could actually hurt you so badly. But it is true. Once you begin to deal with feelings and food and weight by starving, bingeing, or purging, it is very, very hard to stop. And it is very difficult to tell others.

This book is filled with the stories of people who found that sharing their experiences was an important part of their continuing recovery. You will be able to hear first hand how little diets and big pressures can be a dangerous mix. You will see how people can carry very dangerous secrets for a long time before they admit that the secret has taken control of their lives. And you will discover how different people may use very different and healthy ways to give up starving, bingeing, and purging, and try new ways to cope with food, feelings, and weight.

Yes, this book is about many different aspects of anorexia nervosa and bulimia. But most importantly, it is about how you can use the power of trust, guidance, and love to share your concerns, understand and even overcome anorexia nervosa and bulimia.

I

UNDERSTANDING ANOREXIA NERVOSA AND BULIMIA

1 | The Basics

Are you dying to be thin? If the question hits home, stop and think for a moment. How much time do you spend every day thinking about your weight? Maybe you diet in spurts, losing those 10 or 15 or 20 pounds, getting all that praise from the people who are important to you. And then maybe gaining that same weight back over a few months, a year, or more.

If you are like millions of Americans, you fight that battle of the bulge every day. You worry about your belly, chin, thighs, arms, or some other part of your body that you feel bad about because you think it's too fat. And you compare your body to the tight, supple bodies of men and women on television, in movies, and in magazines every day. Then you look in the mirror again, and maybe, just for a moment, all you can see is that part of your body that you hate. You forget that you are much more than a sum of your various body parts, that you do look good, and that you make other people feel good just for being yourself.

Then you move on through your day, thinking about all sorts

of things, including food and your weight. You might have lunch or dinner with family or friends, or maybe you eat alone that day. In either situation, you enjoy the food—the taste, the comfort, the control you can exert as you eat just what you want to eat. You might even continue to eat long after you satisfy your hunger. Then, you might add a dessert to that meal, because you want it. After you finish everything you want to eat, you might feel bloated, annoyed, guilty, angry at other people for letting you eat so much, or angry at yourself. But you also might feel happy because you really enjoyed that food.

As you are feeling these conflicting reactions to the food you have eaten and the weight you might gain, you may think about other people you know who seem to be able to eat anything, in any amount, and still stay thin. At a moment like that, those people seem to have everything, because they seem to be able to have their cake, and eat it, too! And you might feel jealous of that ability to eat whatever and whenever they want, without ever gaining any weight.

Well, bulimia is an eating disorder that can develop from that very feeling of wanting to eat endlessly, without gaining weight. People who are bulimic binge on a wide variety of foods, including highly caloric foods, such as cake, candy, and ice cream. On a schedule that can range from once in a while to several times a day, people suffering from bulimia will secretly buy large quantities of food. Then they will systematically eat as much as they possibly can, until they are literally in agony, or until someone interrupts them. Then they feel an overwhelming need to get rid of all that food they have just eaten. So they may force themselves to vomit. Or they may take laxatives and other drugs to purge themselves of the fluid and solid waste in their bodies.

To eat an enormous amount of food is called bingeing, and to forcibly eliminate that food is identified as the act of purging. The cycle of eating vast quantities of food and then vomiting or using drugs to force that food out of the body is referred to as the ''binge/purge'' cycle.

Where Is the Harm?

Maybe you think that bingeing and purging is a great way to eat what you want and stay thin. Or you may think that purging after a meal will help you lose weight so you can fit into a special outfit for a very special occasion. Before you decide that purging after a binge once in a while is a perfect solution to eating and weighing what you want, you have to understand the facts. Purging is habit forming. In fact, you will learn from bulimic people that bingeing becomes a mere avenue to purging.

Every bulimic begins with just one purge. And then just one more. Then he or she does it again, because it becomes easier with some practice. Bingeing, purging, or both can start as a once-in-a-while means of eating and still wear your prom dress or qualifying for an athletic event, but it can rapidly become a ritual to engage in once, twice, even a dozen times in a week or a day.

If that sounds hard to believe, then focus on this second point: Bingeing and purging can give a person an enormously satisfying feeling of self-control and gratification. After all, he has figured out how to eat whatever he wants and still be free of bad feelings that can come after he eats food that he thinks is ''bad.'' Eventually, that first, wonderful feeling of controlling everything that goes into or out of the body gradually disappears, and the body takes over. The disorder then controls the person.

As you might imagine, bingeing and purging requires elaborate and creative planning, especially when no friend or family member knows. Protecting the secret is as important as the binge/purge process itself. That means that bulimic people can spend days and hours planning strategies to acquire, consume, and then purge their food. While they work, play, talk, watch TV, make love, or accomplish ordinary daily chores, they may be planning when, how, and where to get hold of the food, eat it, and then purge, one way or another. And the people who live, work, play, watch TV, and finish those daily chores with a bulimic friend, colleague, or family member may not have a clue that someone they are so close to is going through this consuming, wrenching process in secret.

Maybe you can see by now that the first harm can come from the lying, manipulation, and secrecy that surrounds bingeing and purging. One of the earliest effects of that whole bulimic cycle is the damage done to relationships as the bulimic focuses on protecting that secret, instead of fostering trust in a friendship or an intimate relationship.

The harmful effects are not limited to the damage done to personal relationships, however. The other major area of harm is physical, and you can understand the basic dangers without knowing anything about medicine or human biology. The human digestive system is basically like a one-way street. In an emergency, you can go the wrong way down that street if absolutely necessary, but it's dangerous to try to go the wrong way on a regular basis. The human digestive process works on the same assumptions: In an emergency, when you have consumed some dangerous substance or spoiled food, it would be logical to force vomiting. Under ordinary conditions, however, the body eliminates liquid and solid waste in an orderly, regular way, so that nutrients are absorbed and waste is discarded. When the body is allowed to go through that digestive process at a normal pace, all the body parts involved can remain in good working order.

When the body is forced to accept vast quantities of food and then is forced to expel that food before it is processed, a huge physical burden develops. If you fail to allow your body to work the way it is designed to function, then the body parts you do not use can begin to show serious signs of trouble. And those first signs can be really ugly. For instance, many bulimics complain that their teeth blacken and begin to fall out, because the acid in their vomit actually corrodes the enamel on their teeth.

Problems with appearance and with dental health can also affect people who suffer from anorexia (self-starvation). On their way to becoming what they think is perfectly thin, they may find themselves losing their hair, even if that hair had always been thick and lustrous. So, young women who are anorexic can suddenly have to cope with getting bald. Then, eyelashes can fall out, and skin can get visibly blotchy, with red and yellowish marks all over. And those are just a few of the problems that can show up on the outside, while the individual person is struggling fiercely to keep that secret deep inside.

Other alarming, dangerous conditions can develop in response to the physical violence done to the body through the binge/purge cycle or through self-starvation. More detailed information is presented in Chapters Two and Three and in the personal accounts shared here by people who decided to tell their stories so that you could learn from their suffering and from their relief in recovery.

At this point, you know key basics about bulimia. People who suffer from bulimia binge and purge, and that binge/purge process can take over and control a person, just like any other addiction. There is one last critical aspect of bulimia that you must understand: *People who are bulimic are not necessarily thin!*

In fact, many bulimics can become somewhat overweight at various times in their lives. Their weight can vary by as much as 10 to 15 pounds over or under a level that is healthy for them, based on age, height, and frame size. Those people who do become very thin, so that they weigh approximately 25 percent less than is good for them because they have intentionally stopped eating, are suffering from anorexia nervosa.

Food and Fear: A Deadly Combination

Anorexia is like many other health problems: It takes time to develop. That means that early signs can be detected, and when those signs lead someone to get professional help as soon as possible, intervention can be very successful. However, anorexia can defy early identification for two very simple reasons.

First of all, the early signs of anorexia can give friends, family, and colleagues encouragement and pleasure. Everyone may be very happy that the person involved is dieting successfully or taking more responsibility for managing his or her food intake. That generally positive feeling can prevail to the point where it is very difficult to see that the person's eating habits are really not appropriate at all.

The second primary reason why it can be difficult to detect anorexia in the very early stages is that the outward changes may develop slowly in the beginning. The medical symptoms of this disorder can be associated with a wide range of disorders, and this fact can lead to a medical wild goose chase lasting weeks, months, even years.

The third basic reason why it can be difficult to identify anorexia in its very early stages is that the first signs are not difficult for the anorexic individual to hide. Weight loss can be concealed in fashionable clothes, and virtual self-starvation can be confused with a short-term diet.

Even though anorexia becomes entrenched only over time, it gathers force as the disorder takes hold. Suddenly, the young girl who was your best friend, your favorite most outgoing student, your most obedient and dependable child, can seem obsessed with food. She might like to prepare it elaborately. She might love to see you eat it. But she no longer eats in a way that can possibly be healthy for her. Her eating habits seem to be the whole focus of her life. And you cannot seem to change her mind, no matter what you do.

Maybe you thought dieting was a good idea at first, because

you felt it was good for her to lose a few pounds and to stay away from all those fattening foods. But the good idea is out of control, and this person who is so important to you, who always was there to do what was expected, seems less and less willing to be the girl you always knew. She seems to have undergone a profound and private change.

That change actually took place right in front of your eyes, and she might seem to enjoy your reaction when it finally becomes clear to you that something is seriously wrong. She may point out that she lost weight because she's supposed to be thin, and she still has more to lose, because she thinks she has a fat face or fat thighs. It may seem that she is fixated on that part of her body and puts all her incredible, boundless energy into dealing with food. In fact, she may appear to be very much afraid of getting fat, even though she is so thin that you cannot find any fat on her body at all. You cannot pinch even a fraction of an inch.

She may let you think that she has eaten something, showing you that she has gained a few pounds and allowing you to feel victorious as a friend, parent, teacher, spouse, or coworker. But in reality, she has not eaten anything substantial at all. She certainly has avoided eating any food that could stay in her body and provide adequate nourishment. She could have sat at the dinner table, proudly pointing out that she ate everything—that she's an official member of the "clean plate club"—while she really fed most of her meal to the dog waiting under the table. Or folded the food into a napkin in the split seconds when no one would notice. Then, she could quickly drink large quantities of water before getting on the scale, so she can point proudly to the weight gain you might start to demand out of concern for her health.

How Dangerous Is Anorexia?

Very simply, anorexia nervosa is self-starvation. It can be

effects of starvation, right in the middle of a family that has always had more than enough food to keep everyone healthy and happy. Anorexia can cause extensive, damaging medical problems that can be highly visible—or very difficult to see. These problems can start with loss of hair and teeth and can move rapidly to discolored skin, chronically swollen glands, kidney dysfunction, liver trouble, heart disturbances, hyper active behavior, and hypotension (low blood pressure).

Can all this start with a simple diet? Yes, if three conditions are in place. First, the individual involved identifies the diet as being absolutely crucial to life success. That means that the person feels nothing good can happen in life until she or he becomes thin enough. So that person concentrates extraordinary energy on the diet, which can become more important than anyone or anything else in the world.

Second, the person persists in stringent dieting, even after achieving a goal that might be considered a healthy weight for that particular individual. And the third early warning sign is the development of very special food rituals. The person may eat but may choose only broiled chicken. Or peanut butter. Or specific, measured amounts of asparagus. Day in and day out.

Does this particular eating disorder affect only girls and women? No. Although the problem generally affects women and pubescent or teenage girls, it does develop in men and boys. Even so, female anorexics outnumber their male counterparts by about 15 to 1. And if they receive good, timely treatment, male anorexics tend to have just one major bout with the illness. Female anorexics are more likely than male anorexics to start a pattern that can dominate their entire lives.

As you absorb the lives of the people affected by anorexia who chose to share their experiences with you, it will become easier for you to get to know the fears and hopes inextricably tied to this particular eating disorder: How hard it is for anorexics to trust, and how they can persist in their efforts to recover. Among those who have contributed their insights here are some who have yet to begin substantive recovery. They have told their stories anyway, because they wanted to help you understand how hard it can be to change—even when the change is admittedly positive.

Taking the Die Out of Dieting

You probably recognize some familiar feelings you might have in common with people who develop anorexia or bulimia. You may say to yourself, "I wish I could have anorexia for just two weeks, so I could take off these ten pounds!"

You may not think about food all the time, the way many anorexic people concentrate on food. In fact, there may be many other things and people you think about more often than food. But you may go through a cycle of denying yourself enough food, eating too much to make up for that period of self-denial, disliking yourself for eating too much, and punishing yourself once again by eating too little. Then you probably start the whole cycle over again, because you feel deprived and hungry.

It's an American cycle, one that produces dancers who are generally ten pounds lighter than those in Europe, athletes who are convinced that their peak performance is impossible without purging, and ordinary young people who feel so powerless and overwhelmed that they turn inward to find a world they can control. Because inside their bodies, they have absolute control. Control over food, family, and everything important to them. Even if that control means they are slowly taking their own lives. It's still their decision, they argue, and that fact can make the whole painful effort seem worthwhile from their point of view. And from their point of view, they cannot quite see that they deserve a life that is free of all the self-inflicted pain and punishment.

You will hear the arguments and witness the process of recovery. That's right: the process of recovery. Just as it can take time for a person to develop anorexia or bulimia, it takes time for that person to go through the recovery process. Anorexic and bulimic people can find change to be just as frightening as anyone else facing the fact that his or her life might have to be altered completely. That fear can make them hold on to the one thing they know, trust and understand: the security and comfort that comes from focusing totally on food.

One by one, we can each help initiate and maintain the process of change. We can even stop destructive behavior from developing at all, if we start by understanding that some people feel safer in pain, because that pain is a familiar place. You will begin to understand that feeling more completely as you integrate the perspectives shared here by those who offer their stories in these pages. With that basic understanding and a working grasp of the key facts presented in this short section, you can become part of the crucial effort to take the "die" out of "dieting."

An Added Note on Another Basic: Bulimarexia

You read it correctly. The word "bulimarexia" is a combination of the words "bulimia" and "anorexia." It describes a combination disorder that involves the seriously low body weight of anorexics and the binge/purge cycle that characterizes bulimia. Many anorexics go through bulimic episodes, and there are bulimics who do become anorexic as their weight drops steeply and they become fearful of being "fat."

The stories that unfold in these pages will help you begin to understand how such eating disorders can develop, and how they can be identified, stopped, and even prevented.

What You Can Do Today

What can you possibly do to help reduce the incidence of these dangerous disorders in your own world? More than you think. For instance, you may know a young girl who is going through puberty right now. She's probably very involved with the physical changes in her body. And if those changes surprise you, imagine how they must surprise her! If that young girl feels that her physical development is somehow ugly, she may believe she can eliminate those changes by dieting away any chance of growing up at all.

Whether you are her father, mother, coach, doctor, counselor, or friend, she may start that diet in an effort to please you. Even if you do not actually tell her in so many words that you want her to lose weight, she may feel that you would love and respect her more if she were thinner. Or that you would notice her more if she could somehow just take charge of something that would capture your attention. She may even feel that starving would protect her from the social and sexual pressures of becoming a woman. And that dieting away all that physical change will save her from the complicated adult world that can be so frightening.

Many situations can contribute to the development of anorexia nervosa, bulimia, or bulimarexia. It is impossible to guess at all the different reasons that may underlie such disorders. However, there is one important and very comforting thing you can keep in mind. It is not necessarily your fault that someone you care about develops such an eating disorder. Too often, books, TV shows, magazine articles, and even some professionals try to place blame on the family. Or the school. Or the media. The point is simple: Blame is not the issue.

Blame can lead to guilt, and guilt can make us feel compelled to keep secrets. Keeping guilty secrets because we feel bad just reinforces the mechanism of the eating disorders, which thrive on that sense of shame. Worst of all, focusing on blame distracts us from the real work of preventing anorexia and bulimia. Trying to assign blame also gets in the way of crucial efforts to identify and treat people and families suffering with the problems of anorexia or bulimia. Anything that gets in the way of that real work can cost lives, and when a life is lost while everyone is trying to assign or take blame, the guilt can become unbearable.

You can see how it is pointless and even dangerous to point fingers. But it *is* important for you to know just how big a role you can play in someone's life when the issues involve self-image and the person's need to please you. Anorexics and bulimics can begin on the path to their disorder by trying to please someone important to them, such as a boyfriend, girlfriend, spouse, parent, or teacher.

In fact, this entire process can begin without any knowledge on your part. This person whom you care about, and who cares about you, can begin by trying desperately to please you and can end up entirely out of control, serving a body that is in revolt and shutting you out completely in the process.

How Does It Happen?

It happens because the disorder helps that individual person achieve a goal. That goal may be to become thinner, more lovable, more in control, or even to reject a sexual identity. It happens behind closed doors, often involving people and families who appear to have everything they could possibly want in life.

We are losing the spirit, the contribution, and even the lives of girls and boys, women and even some men, because of the destructive impact of these eating disorders. But we have a choice. Each one of us can make a difference. And we can start by learning to distinguish the people we love from the things they do for us or for others. And we can stay informed.

Your Role: Part of the Solution

You can be part of the solution, starting right now. You can begin by developing a clear understanding of how anorexia and bulimia develop and how these disorders can involve dangerous medical and psychological complications.

2 | Slender Chances: The Dangers of Anorexia Nervosa

I have a very vivid memory of sitting in fifth grade on the first day of class and feeling totally safe. The sun was streaming in, the classroom was colorful and friendly, and I was on top of the world. Whatever the teacher expected, I understood. Whatever the kids did, I knew how to handle myself. There were no surprises. I was 11 years old, and I could do anything they handed me. For ten years following that day, I kept that image firmly planted in the front of my mind. All through junior high, high school, college, marriage, and two hospital stays, I yearned for that one last year when things were so neatly in place.
—**Ann Frankl, age 22**
Recovering anorexic

Imagine yourself as a young child. Your entire world depends on your parents, teachers, and other caretakers. Before your earliest memory, you developed the ability to grasp what adults expected from you, and then you did what was expected. You've become a star at following the rules, getting the grades, being popular, and generally making everyone feel proud of you. You don't worry about your own feelings very much, because you can see from everyone else's attitude that you are successful. Your parents, teachers, and friends admire and reward you, so you must be successful. You feel sure that the stage is set, because you have refined your ability to read the rules and achieve excellence.

How Anorexia Develops

You can adjust to anything, until you start to hit puberty. This is foreign territory. All your life, you could rely on other people to set the standards for you. Now you have all sorts of feelings and messages coming from every direction, and you start to be afraid. How can you manage to succeed and please people if the rules keep changing? The adults in your life always told you what to expect. Now they're asking you. What do you want to do when you grow up? How are you going to handle the pressure of dating? How will you cope with all the different opportunities available to you?

Your parents and teachers may tell you that you're lucky. You have opportunity! The world is wide open for you. With your ability to achieve, you can make anything happen. But inside yourself, you start to feel consumed with doubt. All your past achievements were accomplished because the rules were clear and your options were limited. Now they are limitless. Now, after a lifetime of never having made a decision that was not first made by an adult, you have to make choices about school, work, socializing, sexual impulses and pressures, and the opportunity to take drugs that are available from every direction. In the middle of all this external change, your body is different, inside and out. When you look in the mirror, all you see is change. And when you sit in class, go to a movie, or sit at dinner, you're aware of restless, confusing feelings that are unfamiliar and decidedly unwelcome.

At this point, you may decide, consciously or subconsciously, that you have to get a handle on the situation. You were successful before; you'll be successful again. All you have to do is focus on an important, respected goal that other people will recognize and that you know you can achieve. You don't want to defy your parents or teachers openly, because they may withhold all that affection and approval they give you when you are cooperative and compliant. So you have to come up with some way of getting control over the situation without doing anything that adults would find totally upsetting. If you can find that route to control once again, you can duplicate those comfortable old feelings of safety that made your childhood such a success.

You start to search for some sort of strategy that will make life more predictable and concrete for you, the way it was while you were in elementary school. At that point, you may decide to take control over the one territory you *have* to make safe: your own body. By focusing on taking control over your body, you can ignore all those complex, conflicting, and confusing changes that take place when you become a teenager.

But you don't even make that decision on your own. You seek ''permission'' from someone important to you. It could be your mother, father, sister, brother, teacher, coach, religious leader—anyone you respect and want to please. You won't go through the pain without that permission, because you have no experience with decision-making, and you feel the need to get approval from someone who cares about you.

That permission does not have to be spelled out in so many words. A coach may comment that you might want to lose some weight, or a boyfriend might say that you would be really perfect if you could just lose a few pounds. Your mother or father may be letting you know that this is the time in your life when you have to start being careful about what you eat and when you eat it, because weight gain may creep up on you silently, without warning. Someone important to you may tease you about how your hips or breasts are getting big, or how your belly is sticking out a little more than is desirable.

Yes, people tease and talk with each other about these things all the time. But if you are a teenager who is looking for permission to take control over your body by setting weight goals and suppressing all that physical and emotional change, then you may take those comments to heart and keep them in your heart as you set, achieve, and redefine weight-loss goals that eventually will make you skeletal.

That is how anorexia nervosa can develop in a young man or woman. It does not have to develop at puberty. It can develop later in adolescence or young adulthood, but it generally begins before the young man or woman is 25 years old. The one thing that you can say with confidence about anorexia is that it is different with each person. Some people who develop anorexia have a history of weight problems, and some do not. Many anorexics are white middle or upper-middle class young women in their teens or early twenties, but some anorexics come from entirely different backgrounds. An increasing number of male and nonwhite adolescents and young adults are diagnosed as anorexic, and the disorder can remain entrenched long after a person reaches the age of 30.

There are a few basic conditions that anorexics do share, however. They all starve themselves, and they all have a profound fear of fat. They will focus so relentlessly on weight loss that they will eventually lose at least 25 percent of their normal body weight. They are not suffering from any other medical disorder or social problem that could be associated with loss of appetite, and they deprive themselves of food despite their constant, gnawing hunger.

As you might well imagine, starvation is not a fact of life that you can live with indefinitely. In fact, up to 15 percent of all anorexics die as a result of medical complications that develop because they are starving. If this surprises you, take a moment to think about all the news reports and TV specials devoted to telling you how starvation kills people in areas of the world where hunger is a persistent fact of life. Starvation causes the same medical problems for people who live in an environment where food is available but remains untouched—the one aspect of the environment that can be managed totally.

Amenorrhea: A Sexual Development

Ann Frankl recalls:

At first, when I didn't get my period, I thought, "Oh, no! I'm pregnant." I couldn't figure out how that could have happened, since I always used birth control, but I was still terrified that I might be pregnant. I was such a mess myself, I could never have been a good mother at that time. Imagine my relief when the doctor said that I had stopped menstruating because I had lost too much weight. I was actually proud! I remember thinking, "How many women in America can lose weight and get rid of the dreaded monthly curse, both at the same time?" Naturally, I kept using birth control, just in case. There was no way I wanted to get pregnant, even though I was married at that time. I didn't want a baby, and neither did my husband, so none of it really mattered to me.

Ann Frankl's feelings about the fact that she had stopped menstruating are fairly typical of young women who become anorexic. It was gratifying for her to control an unpleasant, inconvenient aspect of being female, and she was proud of that achievement. She knew that her period could and would probably start again once she started to eat. Knowing this, she chose to continue starving herself, testing to see what other bodily functions she could control or eliminate by triumphing over her constant hunger, and continuing to starve.

What Happens to Your Breasts

Women's breasts are made up of a certain amount of fat. If a woman begins to starve, she may begin to lose the fat necessary to keep her breasts soft, rounded, and healthy. No matter whether her breasts are large or small, they can become atrophied as a result of starvation. If you can recall seeing the naked breasts of women in photographs and television reports of people starving in countries far away, you can visualize what atrophied breasts can look like: small and withered. For some women who want to eliminate that soft roundness of their breasts, this is a significant reward.

Lauren, a dancer in a major New York City ballet company, told her psychiatrist that her breasts are too large. "I hate it when I get my period," she complained. "I can feel my breasts swelling until I think I will choke to death. I wish my period would just stop."

If you were to look at Lauren, you would know that the smallest bra is too large for her, and the swelling that comes from her occasional period is imperceptible, if there at all. The only reality that counts, however, is her own. From her point of view, her breasts are disfiguring, getting in the way of her career and her beauty.

Starving Puts Hair on Your Chest

It was really strange. My girlfriend's skin was always perfectly smooth and soft. I loved touching her. I had noticed that her skin started to feel different, and in the sunlight on the beach I realized that she had this light layer of hair growing all over the upper part of her torso and her arms and hands—even her face and neck. It wasn't just the peach fuzz that women have. It was odd, but I didn't say anything. I didn't want to make her self-conscious.

Later on, after she got really sick and her parents decided she had to go to a psychologist because her attitude about eating was so weird, I found out that other women with anorexia get that same hairy growth. It's called lanugo, and it's awful. After a while, it will probably go away if you just eat normally, but she really couldn't. She never ate in front of me, even when she cooked me a meal, and she just kept getting thinner and thinner. It was really frightening.

Lanugo does look and feel strange, and Allen Lesko noticed a problem that his girlfriend had chosen to ignore. Once he pointed it out to her, she tried all kinds of ways to hide that growth, but it was hard to show off her thin body on the beach and still hide the new problem.

Long after the relationship had ended, and the young woman had finally sought help to cope with all the confusing feelings she had about taking on adolescence and adulthood, she called her old boyfriend and thanked him for making her admit that her body was beginning to do things she could not control. When he called attention to the problem in a loving and concerned way, she was amazed. He wasn't telling her she was good or bad. He was just concerned. It was the first time she was aware that another person could just respond to her decision-making without trying to control her.

Bald Spots: Losing Your Hair Where It Matters Most

One of the first casualties of starvation is the hair on top of your head. No matter if your hair is strong or weak, shiny or dull, oily or dry, it will start to break and fall out if you starve yourself. Women as well as men find that no conditioner, treatment, or brush will help stem the process. The only way to make your hair bounce back into shape is to nourish your body with the food it needs first to survive, and then to thrive.

When the Heat Is On

Being in a state of starvation makes your body react differently to heat and cold. A father who was proud of the fact that he had designed a home that was temperature-controlled the year round, without anyone ever having to touch the thermostat, could not figure out why his house would be suddenly and unpredictably hot or cold. It soon became clear that his daughter was manipulating the thermostat mechanism to accommodate the fact that she would get so uncomfortably warm or chilly. When the other people in the house were warm, she wasn't, and the whole problem became a serious source of conflict in her house.

The medical expression for her problem is "abnormal thermoregulation." The body's thermostat can be returned to normal once the anorexic person achieves a normal body weight.

"I Can Do That!": The Hyperactivity Connection

Brenda was the most extraordinarily productive young woman I have ever met. She had so much energy, I would get tired just watching her. I had her in my science class for two semesters, before her parents placed her in a residential hospital program because she had broken her promise not to lose any more weight. She was so thin, she could run in between raindrops, and I really think she did.

She would stand to take notes, race around and do errands, help other kids clean up after lab experiments—she was just one little blur from the beginning of class to the end. I asked her other teachers if she was like this all the time, because I really thought she was on some sort of drugs. They said she was the same in their classes, and if the class required that she stay seated, she seemed always poised to fly out of her seat and get something done. Everyone agreed; we wished all the kids were so good, but we also worried. It was as if she was too good to be true. As it turned out, we were right. We just didn't know it was related to her being so desperately thin. You would think that starvation would make people tired, but it seems that just isn't true. I learned that anorexia really does make people hyperactive, but at the same time, I just admired her for all her self-control and productivity.

Louise Vogel taught high school science for twelve years before she met Brenda, who was Louise's first student suffering from overt signs of anorexia. Louise didn't know anything about the disorder, and she had no idea that the things she was admiring and accepting about Brenda were the very things that were to bring her student first to a hospital and finally to outpatient treatment that has continued for the last two years.

What Do You Call It When Your Skin Turns Yellow?

For reasons that are not understood as yet, anorexic people develop skin coloration called hypercarotinemia. That simply means that if you starve yourself, your skin will become noticeably yellow over time. It's one more aspect of anorexia that you just cannot keep secret, no matter how many layers of clothing you wear, or how much makeup you put on. Some part of your skin will show, and it will be noticed. Then you have to cope with the questions about what it is that is making you develop yellowed skin, in addition to the other physical problems, like loss of hair, increased hair on your torso and extremities, and trouble controlling your impulse to jump up and keep moving, even when everyone else is sitting still.

When Anorexics Binge and Purge

In addition to their own special medical problems that develop as a result of starvation behavior, anorexics often develop the physical symptoms and difficulties experienced by bulimics. These medical problems, such as electrolyte (blood chemical) imbalance and ulcer conditions, occur when anorexics binge and purge as part of their unsuccessful efforts to cope with the pain of hunger and still control their weight. For more explicit information about the medical problems that develop from bingeing and purging, turn to Karen's story in Chapter Four. The information relates to *every* anorexic who may be either bingeing or purging in any way.

Gaining on the Enemy

Being anorexic, like being bulimic, means that you are at war with your own body. If you plan to win, what will you gain, and what will you lose? If you win over your body, you must ask yourself whether you will still have a body to control. You can decide to win in cooperation with your body, and then you can be here to enjoy your victory. The first step comes when you decide to stop focusing on food and start focusing on your feelings. If your problem is bulimia, it is equally important to stop emphasizing all the issues of food and start looking at feelings.

3 | Why Bulimia Is So Destructive

> I remember thinking, hey, other people lose weight this way, and they lead good lives, like actresses and dancers and athletes. I figured, if they can do it and look that good, so could I. Now I know that you don't hear the whole story when people come out looking so great. Those people put a good front on for the camera. The real story stays the way it was for me: behind closed doors. Until someone smart enough and strong enough helps you discover that you're killing yourself.
>
> —Barbara Orlando, age 36
> **Recovering bulimic**

Bulimia is not a new, improved way to diet. It's a primary disorder that gets progressively worse without treatment. The medical term "primary disorder" means bulimia is not a symptom of something else more fundamental. It is a disorder in itself. It can be accurately diagnosed and successfully treated. But without the right care, bulimia can and will become progressively worse, as the bulimic person feels an increasingly intense compulsion to binge and then purge.

You may feel that it's harmless enough to just eat what you like and then either vomit or use drugs to get rid of what you ate. If you have to weigh in at a diet center or reach a weight goal you have set all by yourself, you may think you can balance overeating with purging. The problem is that you never get balance that way. You get imbalance. That biochemical imbalance, combined with the violence to the digestive process, conspire to produce physical effects that can range from disfiguring to fatal.

Good Food, Bad Food: How Much Is Too Much?

Jason Powell recalls:

All I had to do was eat one cookie, and I would start feeling guilty for eating the wrong thing. Basically, I would feel so guilty, I would just give in and eat the whole box. After all, who cared? From my point of view, a miss was as good as a mile. Once I ate even a little food like candy or cookies or cake or pizza, it was all over. I would eat until I was in pain, or until there was no more food. Then I would start thinking about how much I had eaten, and I would panic. I had to get rid of all that food, so I would make myself throw up.

Before Jason could get control over the bingeing and purging, he had to better understand the concept of portions. Like most other bulimics, Jason had difficulty differentiating between large and small amounts of food, and he focused considerable attention on labeling foods either good or bad. Once he would eat even a bit of "bad" food, he would feel that he had committed a violation of the high standards he had set for himself. He could not see that one cookie was different from a box of cookies, so he would continue to consume the food until he could not eat any more, or until there was no more food.

From Binge to Purge:
The Violent Compulsion

The impulse to indulge in a food the person has labeled "bad" can be the single action that starts the bulimic episode. Like Jason, that person can feel so guilty for having consumed all those forbidden calories that forced vomiting seems to be the only choice. People who develop bulimia do not see that they are capable of small lapses in judgment. To them, there is no such thing as a moderate amount of a food they have labeled "bad."

Once the vomiting is complete, bulimic people can feel a genuine sense of relief. All the bloated, fat, embarrassed, guilty, and angry feelings that were part of the binge disappear. Erin Palmer describes her first purge as one of the most rewarding moments of her life before she entered therapy:

The whole purge process was cleansing. It was a combination of every type of spiritual, sexual, and emotional relief I had ever felt in my life. Purging became the release for me. First, I felt a tremendous rush that you could really call orgasmic. Then, I relaxed completely and fell asleep. After a while, I was hooked. I actually believed that I had to purge to just fall asleep.

Getting hooked is exactly what happens. The purging process and aftereffects can be so completely gratifying for the bulimic that he or she can become totally focused on repeating that same intensely rewarding experience. To achieve a successful episode of vomiting without having to try too hard to vomit, bulimic people will eat as much as possible. If they consume only a small amount of food, vomiting can be difficult.

Once the bulimic person feels the need to purge, then it is necessary for him or her to binge. At that point in the progression of the disorder, a binge may be precipitated not by guilty feelings for having eaten a "bad" food but by the clear and focused need to expel food and feel the expected relaxation effect. The food may still be primarily or exclusively high-carbohydrate, high-sugar desserts like candy, cake, or ice cream, but the focus of the compulsion is on filling the stomach up to the point that it is easier to purge.

For those of us who have never chosen to vomit in order to feel emotional or physical gratification, it can be difficult to understand this whole process. Suppose you are not bulimic. If you were to list words describing the feelings before, during, and after vomiting, you would probably not use "orgasmic," "eager," or "wonderfully relaxed."

If your experience with vomiting is limited to some bouts of the flu or food poisoning, then you may think that it's impossible for anyone to actually want to purge. However, the reality is that people who suffer from bulimia genuinely look forward to the feeling. Medically, the purge may affect chemicals in the brain called neurotransmitters, causing the individual to feel the postpurge gratification most bulimics experience. Medical research into this possibility continues. At this time, however, the impact that purging has on neurotransmitters is still uncertain.

Whether the bulimic individual experiences the surge or rush as a result of emotional, physical, biochemical, or psychological factors, or as a consequence of a combination of those factors, the fact remains that bulimic people often develop a need to experience the feelings of relief associated with purging. Ultimately, they can believe that purging is their only hope of relaxing or feeling complete.

Why Purging Doesn't Help You Lose Weight

Purging can seem harmless enough at first, especially if it makes a person feel good, and it keeps the calories away. Many people ask, "How bad can it be to purge after eating too much?'' The answer is that it can be very bad. Worst of all, the bad effects can develop at different times for different people, so there are no guarantees. Much of the damage takes place inside, so it can be near impossible to tell how bad the problems are until they are very far advanced. By that time, the bulimic person can be as dependent on bingeing and purging as an addict can be dependent on a drug.

The progression of the disorder and the dependency can be understood very clearly. Most bulimic people start purging after a binge, in order to lose or control weight. At first, the bingeing and purging may seem to accomplish that goal. After all, if you weigh yourself in the morning, weigh yourself after a binge, and then weigh yourself again after a purge, you will clearly lose weight. The problem is that most of the weight is water and will naturally come back. The person gets locked into a cycle of checking the scale continuously through the day, feeling great success when it shows weight loss and great anger and shame when it shows any gain.

Bernadette Rogers remembers how desperate she began to feel when the scale showed that she was beginning to gain weight:

I couldn't believe it! There I was, not keeping anything in my stomach for more than half an hour, and sometimes I would only chew my food and not swallow it at all. I would pretend that I was using my napkin to wipe off my mouth, but I would really just chew the food, and then hide it in my napkin. I did that at home for months, and no one ever noticed. Even on days when I didn't purge or binge, I would just chew my food, or not eat at all. That way, I thought I was making up for calories I took in from holding the food in my stomach for a little while. At first, I was able to knock off weight really fast. Then, I realized that I was gaining, even with everything I was doing. Now that I've been going to Dr. Zimmer, I understand what was happening.

* * *

What was happening is a simple fact of human survival. Food digestion begins the moment food goes into the mouth and saliva glands begin the process of digesting and absorbing foods. When a person starves, either continually or for limited periods of time, the body starts to conserve calories. The body's metabolism slows down, so calories are burned off more slowly. At this time, the body will also try to absorb every single bit of nutrition possible.

As soon as the bulimic person puts food into his or her mouth, the salivary glands start to either absorb or predigest that food. Since bulimic people do not absorb enough nutrition through the normal digestive process, the salivary glands take on a more significant role. Bulimic people will often experience dramatic swelling of the salivary glands that leads to "chipmunk cheeks"—enlarged cheeks or jowls.

Those enlarged salivary glands absorb or predigest every bit of food possible. With increasingly active salivary glands and a significantly decreased basal metabolism, the bulimic person may even experience weight *gain,* despite avoiding regular meals and purging without fail after every binge.

Once the bulimic person gets on the scale and sees the increase in weight, he or she may look for new ways to lose weight or maintain enough weight loss to feel successful. "When I couldn't stay at just 150 pounds, I panicked," recalls Marty Brenner. "Then I told myself that if I was smart enough to figure out a way to have my cake and eat it, too, then I was smart enough to find new ways to purge that food that was staying in my body. That's when I started taking laxatives and diuretics. As soon as I started taking those, I could guarantee that my scale would read the right weight. For a while, anyway."

Marty's pattern of moving from one type of purge behavior to another is very common. At first, it can make the bulimic person lose weight, according to the scale. But that scale is deceptive. It doesn't tell you how fat you are. It just tells you how much you weigh.

Laxatives help you empty about a third of the colon at a time. Then it takes time for the body to build up enough waste to fill the colon again, so the bulimic person who is not eating enough to fill that colon will get anxious about being constipated and will use the laxative again. The only way to break the cycle of laxative use and constipation is to stop using the laxatives and to eat foods that will help fill the colon and then allow the colon to function properly.

Diuretics ("water pills") help flush fluid from your body. While certain temporary or chronic physical conditions may make it necessary to use diuretics to process body fluids, bulimia is not one of those conditions. Diuretics simply serve to purge the system of precious fluid while the bulimic continues to intentionally deprive himself or herself of proper fluid intake.

Just as laxative abuse can ultimately lead to constipation and dehydration problems, diuretic abuse also leads to dehydration. The lack of fluids in the system compels the bulimic to drink large quantities of fluids, which then help push the scale up when the bulimic weighs in. The higher weight reading alarms the bulimic, who then purges with laxatives, diuretics, and/or vomiting. Then the dehydration and constipation set in, and the cycle is repeated. The only way to arrest that process is to stop using the diuretics, allow the fluid to build up in the system at a natural rate, and then release those fluids when the pressure develops naturally.

Simply eating and drinking properly and waiting for the body to process the food and fluids properly may seem like the logical way to cope with hunger, food, and nutrition, but the active bulimic finds nothing simple about eating. He or she may feel a driving, overwhelming need to gain control over weight loss through bowel movement or induced vomiting on demand. Without purging, the bulimic person may literally panic. Bulimia often develops in people who feel the need to assert maximum control over their lives, their weight, and/or their bodily functions. That crucial sense of being in control is threatened by the constipation or fluid buildup. It is secured once again through the laxatives and diuretics.

Clearly, the violent compulsion to binge and purge involves medical and psychological dynamics that can vary from person to person. Some of these dynamics are not yet fully understood. The one thing that can be said with certainty is that bingeing and purging is a vicious cycle with insidious medical effects that are difficult to identify when bulimia is in its early stages. However, you can learn to identify those physical signs, which can start with a trip to the dentist.

Smile Appeal: An Early Casualty of Bulimia

I can honestly say that the first thing I noticed about my wife was that she had a gorgeous smile. It was dazzling. I fell in love with her for all sorts of reasons, but that smile was the first thing that caught my eye. And I never took it for granted. I always loved to make her laugh, because her whole face lit up, and her teeth were absolutely perfect. In fact, she was perfect in every way you can think of—pretty, bright, great figure. And a dazzling smile. So you know I would notice when her teeth started to look kind of gray.

I told her I was worried, but she told me it was because she bought the wrong toothpaste. Well, three brands of toothpaste later, her teeth still looked darker. And she refused to go to the dentist. I couldn't believe it! The resistance she put up was so odd—she would make appointments and then cancel them, using some excuse that something urgent was happening at work or home, and she couldn't make the appointment. She was always really sensible and loving, so I never really thought that she was avoiding going to the dentist.

Now I know that the bulimia was destroying her teeth, and the dentist could really have helped, if only we had gone in time. Now, Debra's got to get her teeth all filed down and capped, which is costing us a tremendous amount of money...If only she had gotten to the dentist earlier, we could have saved so much heartache and suffering.

Debra Hillman's husband, Nick, still has difficulty understanding how his wife could consume and purge vast quantities of food over years of marriage without his ever having noticed that anything was wrong. He offered to share his feelings with you, because he felt so frustrated. He was frustrated with himself for having missed something his wife was going through, even though she took great pains to keep her bulimia a secret. Even more to the point, Nick remains frustrated and angry that he chose to just assume everything was really okay, instead of choosing to confront his wife about the fact that she seemed to be avoiding dental appointments and routine checkups.

Nick understands that he had no information or frame of reference to foresee that Debra was avoiding getting help. He never anticipated that Debra was hurting herself, because he could never imagine that she could be unhappy about herself. He adored her, and thought she was perfect. It never occurred to him that perfection was an impossible burden, even though Debra took that burden on herself. Nick was attracted to Debra partly because of her physical beauty and social skills, which he admired but could never match. He never felt as good as Debra, and never imagined that Debra could be dissatisfied with herself in any way.

It's easy to understand how Nick felt, and continues to feel. He keeps wondering what could have happened if his wife had gone to a dentist who could have expressed informed concern about the fact that the enamel on her teeth was actually eroding. Nick believes that one timely confrontation could have motivated Debra to get the help she needed, and Debra believes he is right. On more than one occasion, she has pointed out that she could have avoided so many marital, emotional, physical and medical problems if she had only gone to a doctor who could have understood what was happening to her teeth, and to the rest of her body.

Modern dentistry is interested in ensuring that every reader understand that your dentist can identify dental effects of bulimia. He or she can often provide you with information about the disorder, since dentists are often specifically trained to recognize that bulimia may be indicated when there is etching of the tooth enamel.

That etching can develop because the [regurgitated] stomach acid erodes the hard enamel that protects the dentin, which is the softer inner material of the tooth. If the dentin is exposed and left unprotected, the teeth undergo accelerated wear and are particularly vulnerable to decay. In other words, without extensive capping, bulimia can destroy a beautiful smile. Even with that capping, advanced gum disease can make the patient require dentures.*

The appeal of a bright, healthy smile is what brought Debra and Nick Hillman together. The destruction of that smile, the countless deceptive games Debra played to keep her secret from her husband, and her husband's confusion about the many symptoms Debra began to display, nearly broke their marriage apart.

According to Nick, his family was able to stay together because Debra's serious problems with an inflamed esophagus brought her to the attention of a doctor who had been trained to identify bulimia. Until the doctor diagnosed his wife's illness, Nick just kept trying to act as if everything were okay. He thought that he could make his wife well, and still hold on to all the things that he found important, if he could just keep on behaving as if he and Debra were just fine. The changes in his wife caused him so much anxiety that he started to tell himself there weren't any changes at all—it was all his imagination. He tried to hold on to that feeling, until a doctor helped Debra and

---

*Dr. Joseph Vitale, practitioner of general dentistry

Nick accept the reality that her intensely painful condition of esophagitis was caused by her constant vomiting.

The Searing Pain of Esophagitis

Pain is a regular part of the day when you are bulimic. Part of the enormous satisfaction you derive from your struggle with food is that you win over pain and denial. Some of that pain is related to the fact that the vomiting associated with bulimic behavior can irritate the esophagus, and lead to esophagitis.

If you check the dictionary, you will find that the esophagus is "the tube through which food passes from the pharynx [throat] to the stomach." When you are bulimic, the food travels both ways in a violent assault on the whole digestive process. The esophagus was meant to carry food down on a regular basis, and up only in an emergency. The purging reverses the natural order of things and can bring on medical effects even more painful and disruptive than esophagitis.

From Pain to Danger: When the Esophagus Bursts

There is only so much stress and irritation that the esophagus can endure before it actually bursts apart, or ruptures. People who suffer a ruptured esophagus may survive after hospitalization and extensive, delicate surgery. However, the digestive system can be permanently damaged by the destruction that can begin with one single episode of vomiting to fit into some special clothing, participate in sports, or cope with feelings of anger and helplessness.

It is crucial for you to know that there is no way to tell when a person has reached the point where his or her esophagus could burst from the incredible acidity and pressure that are part of vomiting. Some people can develop a life-threatening ruptured esophagus after having been bulimic for only a short time, while others can develop the same symptoms after longer periods of time. There is no way to control the extent of the damage done by your stomach acid, and it is impossible to reduce the violent nature of regurgitation. Without warning, a ruptured esophagus can permanently damage your health. It can even cost you your life.

Stress Ulcers: Not a Matter of Age

The hardest thing for me to face was that the food rituals I followed religiously to get control over my body ultimately put my body on the losing side of an internal war that was completely beyond my understanding. So it was completely beyond my control. There I was, so proud of regulating my weight right down to the ounce. I was the only guy on the wrestling team who could accomplish exactly the weight the coach set. And there I was, sitting doubled over in the doctor's office, lying to him. Telling him I never spit up blood, and I just had a stomachache from my lunch.

Being an important member of the wrestling team was just one of the many things Dan Parnyc could point to with pride. Dan was accomplished at swimming and gymnastics, and he was always on the Dean's List in high school. Now, on the wrestling team in college, he learned that many of his teammates controlled their weight by purging, then made up for it by bingeing, even on days when there was a match. They would share ideas about how to lose weight, or gain weight, as fast as possible. Dan never asked if anyone ever got sick. They all looked fine to him. He felt that, if he was strong enough, he could compete just like the rest. What Dan did not realize was that many of his teammates had been to their own doctors, with complaints about abdominal pain or other pain-related problems. Once Dan had gone through a complete physical examination, his doctor ordered him to get a series of gastrointestinal tests known as an "Upper GI" to determine whether he had an ulcer. Much to his surprise, Dan was told that he did have a small stress ulcer and that he would have to be very careful about what he ate.

I was upset that something like an ulcer could happen inside me without me even knowing, but I never said that to the doctor. He asked me if I had any questions, after he went through the whole list of good foods and bad foods, and I told him I couldn't think of any. I had the food lists that could beat his coming and going, and I told him I knew all that stuff, and anyway, I didn't think having an ulcer was so bad. Look at all the executives and high-performance type people who have ulcers and look fine.

Well, that was the wrong thing to say. He told me flat out that an ulcer is an open sore on the mucous membrane that is the lining of the intestine. The tissue of the membrane actually disintegrates, and while this hole is being burned inside you, the sore can have pus—Ugh. It was disgusting, just listening to him. I went home and stood in front of the mirror naked. I couldn't believe that a hole was burning inside me, if I could still look like any athlete in top form. I don't mean to brag, but I really looked good. So I started telling myself that the doctor was crazy, and I went out. At the end of that Saturday night, I was hospitalized in incredible pain after my buddy found me throwing up blood in the men's room at the bar.... The next day, a hospital social worker who used to wrestle confronted me about the bulimia. I didn't admit it at first, but the pain and blood from the ulcer really scared me, and I gave in and admitted it to him. I always thought I would be able to stop whenever I wanted, but it was hard. Damned hard. I couldn't control the thing I was doing to take control, which was very confusing. But I'm recovering. I haven't binged or purged in four months.

* * *

Sometimes a frightening, painful medical problem can be a catalyst in helping the bulimic face the reality that he or she *is* bulimic. However, many other people who binge and purge will undergo extensive, painful, costly, and time-consuming medical tests and treatments without ever admitting that the medical problems they are suffering are related to the bingeing or to the different ways and drugs they use to purge.

Dan still feels that he would never have told anyone about the bulimia if the hospital social worker had not faced him with so much solid evidence and insight into the problem. Yes, Dan denied it at first. But he learned to trust that one person, only to discover that he could finally gain control over what happened to his body by stopping the bingeing and purging, and allowing himself to heal.

Potassium, Sodium, and Other Matters of the Heart

Since bulimic people can consume and then purge themselves of anywhere from 5 to 10 pounds of food in a single episode, it may not surprise you that they often suffer problems with their digestive system or dental health. You may know people who appear to live reasonably satisfying lives despite such health problems as ulcers, bad teeth, or unhealthy gums, so long as those people get the right medical care. But the medical effects of bingeing and purging reach beyond gastrointestinal problems to affect the heart.

Harriet remembers:

Lying in the cardiac care unit, I was only vaguely aware of the people around me. I was completely focused on the machines, the tubes, the monitors—everything giving sounds and readouts reflecting what was happening in my body. I remember wishing that I had my own monitor that could help me get control of my body, just like those hospital machines. Even when I was close to dying, I never admitted to anyone that I was bulimic. Not anyone. I can't tell you what I went through, because I can't remember it all. All I know is that I lied like crazy, and they decided that my cardiac arrythmia was attributable to the fact that I was not eating or sleeping properly, and that I had no healthy way of coping with stress. They put me on medication and a diet, with directions about good foods and bad foods, and they made me agree to a rigid exercise regimen. When I left that hospital, the only thing I learned was that I had to get more proficient at balancing my levels of potassium and sodium —all those electrolytes. I never paid a minute's worth of attention to their warnings that I could die if I didn't change. I really felt that I would rather die than change.

Cardiac arrythmia is an irregular heartbeat, and it can kill you. Harriet had no congenital cardiac dysfunction or heart disease. She had caused her heart problems by bingeing and purging. The tremendous violence done to her system caused her to suffer serious electrolyte abnormalities that, in turn, made her heart beat irregularly. When Harriet discovered that the electrolyte imbalance was the trigger mechanism for her episode with cardiac arrythmia, and that the imbalance was causing her to suffer from low blood pressure, she was placed on potassium and sodium and chloride supplements.

At that time, the entire concept of a dietary supplement eluded Harriet. Dietary supplements are designed to do exactly what the name implies: supplement diet. They can work only as catalysts to help the body utilize food, but they do not and cannot replace food.

As soon as they let me out of the hospital, I started to study about electrolytes and nutrition. I bet I knew more than the doctors, I read so much. And I figured that I would be able to control the low blood pressure and the cardiac problems. Looking back now, I can't believe I actually thought that I could maintain my health without ever completely digesting any food.

After my second hospitalization, my sister gave me Dr. Zimmer's telephone number. She said she got it from a girl who was going to him because he was helping her control her bulimia. I remember thinking, "This is just another doctor I can wrap around my finger." Thank God, I was wrong. I haven't binged or vomited or anything in 7 months and 11 days, and I feel so proud!

First, Harriet tried to use her grave illness as a new way to explore even more elaborate tricks to try to control her weight and her body. After her second stay in the cardiac unit, Harriet was still resistant, still denying that anything was wrong. Her original motivation for seeking further medical or psychological care was to find out more tricks that would help her continue to binge and purge. She is alive today because she decided to consider the alternatives. She chose to take the focus off food, to start talking with her therapist about her feelings instead.

Harriet still has lapses. She still chooses to binge and purge occasionally, when the stress in her life builds up, and she loses track of the fact that she can vent that stress by calling a friend, visiting someone, exercising, going to a movie—anything that she may find relaxing and enjoyable. Every time she binges and purges, she knows she is damaging the precious biochemical and digestive balance so crucial to her physical and emotional well-being. The good news is that Harriet can go months without lapsing into a bulimic episode, and she is beginning to understand that she does not destroy all her hard work just because she has a lapse.

As an afterthought, Harriet points out that she is finally healing physically, as well as emotionally.

One of the most amazing things is how much better I feel physically. I used to think I was a superior person if I could tolerate pain, discomfort, and physical or medical problems.

Now that I've been able to abstain for so long, I can see how many different physical problems I was having when I was bingeing and purging. It's hard for me to believe I actually lived in so much pain.

The Headlines Are True

More and more personal stories are being written about and by people who have secretly binged and purged until they become very ill, or until they go for treatment. If you are bulimic, and you do not choose to go for help on your own, your body will force you to go. And if you ignore your body, then you may discover too late that you have to make peace with your body if you expect to live.

If you ignore warning signals that you or someone you care about is bulimic, then you may have to face the development of kidney failure, a burst esophagus, or a ruptured large or small intestine. What do all those medical crises have in common? They can each kill you.

How Much of This Really Happens?

All the medical problems listed above can happen to anyone who is bulimic. Symptoms vary, but the physical problems are inevitable and scary. A compulsion to binge and then purge develops just like a compulsion to take a drug. As soon as you start to binge and purge, your body struggles continuously to maintain some equilibrium, or balance, despite the constant assault on its ability to process food properly.

Paula Mondell remembers reading everything she could get her hands on about the physical problems that can develop because of bulimia.

I remember thinking that if I could only gather all the information possible, I would be able to keep the electrolytes in balance, handle the low blood pressure, deal with the destructive stomach acid by taking antacids....So I read everything, and I knew more than some of the doctors who were supposed to be treating me.

I would go to the chiropractor to handle the lower back pain I would get from bending over the toilet so much, and I would decide to skip using the medications that would help me vomit. Instead, I would stick things down my throat, because I thought it was better for me than the chemicals.

After I would binge, I felt so bloated and disgusting....Then I would vomit or purge some other way, and it would make me feel like a new person. I could fall asleep, cook the perfect meal, dress like a doll—anything I had to get done. It didn't matter that my stomach would hurt like hell, sometimes for hours. It didn't matter that I was losing energy and wasn't strong enough to do the work I always did without any problem. If I was fatigued or stressed, I would just lose myself in the whole vicious cycle—shopping, gorging myself, and then flushing my body free of everything I hated. The pain and the physical problems just didn't matter.

There was one thing that I didn't anticipate. My face got fatter. And it was round to begin with. My boyfriend started calling me "Chipmunk Cheeks," and I hated it. The more I hated it, the more he would make fun of me. Later on, I found out that the bulimia makes your salivary glands get larger and larger, so your body can get some nutrition and fluid as soon as your food goes into your mouth. Those salivary glands puff up inside your mouth, and show up outside, so there you are—chipmunk cheeks! I remember looking in the mirror, about four weeks after I stopped purging, and shouting for joy. "The chipmunk cheeks are gone! Hurray!"

When You Can't Win for Losing

If you are bulimic, then you are caught up in a war where the rules keep changing. You start by trying to take control over your body—what goes in, what goes out, when, and how much are all up to you. You get to feel powerful, knowing that you can have what you crave and still not suffer dreaded weight gain that other people may see. You purge because purging is cleansing. You no longer feel disgusted for having eaten so much. You feel elated for having enjoyed the best of both worlds: the joy of eating anything until you burst, and then expelling everything inside that feels ugly and embarrassing. That feeling of control is virtually intoxicating.

There is just one problem. Your body will give you a good fight. Your body has its own control and survival strategies, and they have nothing to do with purging. They have to do with hanging on for dear life. So, while you first binge and then purge your body of fluids and solid foods, your body is busy holding on to every calorie and every drop of fluid it can find. Eventually, it will take over the decision-making for you by shutting down or disabling parts of your system that demand balanced acid levels, electrolytes, solid food intake, and fluids. That includes your whole body, from head to toe.

If you are bulimic, you may think you can win this fight if you just know enough tricks to keep on losing weight or staying thin, no matter how much you eat. When Janice Baker finally learned that she had done permanent damage to her own liver, she sat quietly in the doctor's office, feeling as if nothing were quite real.

I remember feeling so angry, I was shaking. The doctor left the office to get me a sedative. I mean, I was furious. My body was the one thing I could really manage precisely, and now it was managing me. It was making me make choices, and that made me feel like I was living inside a foreign territory where the environment was really hostile.

At that moment, I felt completely defeated, and I remember saying to my doctor, "I just can't win for losing," and he said to me, "You finally understand. You really can't win if all you want to do is lose." That one comment got us talking for an hour. He was very clear and direct, and talking at that time made me feel better. He wasn't upset by anything I said. He just kept asking me to consider different things. Some of those things were pretty unforgettable. Through that hour, and over the months to come, I kept one thing in the front of my mind: If I get caught up in fighting with my body, I'll lose no matter what. Because my body will fight for a while, and that will be hard to control. And when my body finally stops fighting the war, I'll lose again. Because I'll be the only casualty.

Some of the problems that come from bulimia develop because of the bingeing. Other difficulties develop as a result of vomiting, and then using laxatives or diuretics to purge. Medical complications can be directly or indirectly related to the bulimia, and sometimes it's hard to tell whether your body is having any negative reactions at all. Many of the medical problems can develop silently, until the day they finally explode.

If all this sounds alarming, then you are beginning to really understand that bulimia is not just another way to diet. It can be a painful, isolated way to live, and an awful way to die, but there are choices. Bulimia and anorexia are painful and deadly self-punishments that the victim can learn to understand, control, and eventually overcome.

II

OVERCOMING ANOREXIA NERVOSA AND BULIMIA: THE PRIVATE STORIES

4 | Narrow Escape: Karen's Story

It takes enormous courage and motivation for an anorexic person to open the door to her private life and share her secrets. Karen Anderson had that motivation, because she agreed that you would better understand anorexia if you could hear the private stories of how people can develop such an eating disorder, and how they can learn to recover. Each anorexic person experiences some emotional or physical processes that are unique and some that are common to most people with the same eating disorder, so it is important to understand that Karen's story may or may not include certain phases or experiences that are familiar to you.

At the age of 29, Karen can say that she is a survivor. On her own and self-supporting, she is just beginning to believe that she can establish traditions and routines that do not include the pain and punishment of anorexia. If you were sitting next to her right now, you could see her lean back in her chair and draw deeply on her cigarette, inhaling and then expelling the smoke high into the light that illuminates the room from the corner above her head. With her free hand, she winds a strand of long, dark hair around one finger, carefully considering what she will say because she knows that you will be reading her words.

First, you have to know about being fat. The first thing everyone notices about you is that you're fat. I know, because I was fat from the time I was little. I mean, I was on a diet when I was seven years old. I can honestly say I was fat all my life.

And all my life, whenever I wished for anything, I wished to be skinny. I just knew that if I was skinny, all my problems would be solved. I would be beautiful. I wouldn't have to be afraid—I could be just what I wanted. And I could be what everyone else wanted, too. Let me tell you, being fat is the biggest stigma you can possibly have. Because fat people don't give each other love and support like minorities give each other. Even alcoholics give each other more moral support.

Basically, when you're fat, you're on your own. And I know how everyone thinks about fat people, because I've been on both sides.

I can say this with absolute confidence. You can take the most sophisticated, intelligent, sensitive, perceptive people—and if those people are really honest, they'll tell you that when they see a fat person they think less of her or him than they do of someone who is thin. They think, well, that person doesn't have good self-control. Or they think that someone thin is automatically smarter and better. Because they appear to be able to control what they eat.

I know exactly how thin people feel, too. Because I hear them now. They talk about fat people in front of me now, because I'm so thin. They think they can say anything and that I'll agree with them, because they can see as plain as day that I am thin. So they assume I think that fat people are disgusting slobs.

I don't let them get away with it, I can tell you that. And I knew all my life that people treated me differently because I was fat. My family, friends, teachers, the people I saw at parties and in town—they would act more lenient, or patronizing. But most of all, they were self-important. Showing off how thin they were. Yes. They were self-important. And, I think, just a little sadistic.

Now, you see, I'm unique. I am one of the few people in the entire country who is actually too thin! And I love it! I love it when people see me in a bathing suit, or maybe in the dressing room at a department store. People I don't even know. They come up to me, and they say, "Wow, I can't believe how thin you are!" And some people ask me how I did it.

Well, I'll tell you exactly how I did it. I decided that I was sick of being fat. It was such an effort! I had to work so much harder than skinny people, just to keep up with them. Like when I was fifteen, and I had a boyfriend. I remember everyone saying, "Isn't that nice? Even though she's fat—she actually has a boyfriend!" And you know they're thinking the guy must be really hard up, or that I must be having sex with him, and the really lovable girls don't like him enough to do it with him. And you can't tell me now that people don't say those things, because I'm finally skinny, and I hear how skinny people talk. I was right about everything when I was fat. I knew I had to work harder, run faster, just because I was the fat kid.

And the fat kid grew up to be a fat woman. Then, everyone would tell me, "You would be so pretty if you just lost some weight. You could get married if you just lost some weight." And when I got married despite the fact that I didn't lose any weight, it was like they were disappointed. So they started saying that I would just have to accept that my husband would be cheating on me if I stayed so fat. Hey, I was 200 pounds! They were right!

So I decided it wasn't worth all the extra work. Worrying about my husband. Trying to please my family by being the perfect daughter, putting up with everybody's crap so they would like me, because why else would they like a fat girl? I figured, it's too much work to keep on trying to be so nice. Being skinny would be my ticket to being in charge, for once in my life. I would be free! No more bowing and scraping to everybody!

So far, you can see that weight was the pivotal feature in Karen's life. From her point of view, every accomplishment or failure was related to the fact that she was overweight. The lessons she learned from school and from home reinforced her impression that she had to be better than everyone else at everything possible, because her weight was an inherent social handicap. No one seemed interested in accepting her unless she demonstrated extraordinary mastery. Since her childhood world told her that her weight problem was proof that she could not master her own body, she had to quickly learn how to master pleasing people in other ways. So she was a very well behaved and academically successful child, terrified of open rebellion that could make people reject her completely.

After spending her childhood and adolescence trying desperately to please her parents, teachers, and friends, she discovered that marriage was just a new forum for anxiety and self-doubt. According to her friends and the many television shows and radio programs she heard, her husband was likely to pursue other women unless she made herself more attractive. It was not enough that he had married her. She did not believe that he loved her. She never really felt loved by anyone. She only felt valued by others according to how perfect she could become. Imperfection brought the threat of rejection, so it was better and easier to try to be perfect, hoping to hold on to people who were important.

Finally, Karen felt overwhelmed by all the effort it took to please everyone. She could see that other people were not perfect, and they were loved. The only difference she could see between them and herself was that she was overweight. Following her logic, she firmly believed that she could relax and be herself if she was thin, because she believed that thin people were lovable, and therefore able to concentrate on pleasing themselves, not others.

You already know that Karen could accomplish goals that other people found difficult. She could get superior grades in very difficult subjects, and she could always behave perfectly, even when she was very angry or unhappy. Her history of tightly controlling even her most intense feelings gave her the practice she needed to withstand the pain of hunger and starve herself into what she thought would be the freedom of being thin.

I began to starve myself the same way I did everything else. I wanted to see if I was good at it. So one day I decided to see how many days I could go without eating anything at all. Just drinking some juices. And not eating anything. My mother and father were coming to visit, and they hadn't seen me in almost a year. We had moved out of state, and they were coming up to visit us for two weeks. That was when I decided, hey, wouldn't it be great if I could really make myself thin?

I went five days without eating anything. Just drinking water and a little juice. Let me tell you, I was proud of that. I still am. Of course, at the end of those five days, I was also crazy. My husband took one look at me shaking in the bathroom when I was trying to brush my teeth, and he announced that this was no way to lose weight. But he said it was good that I wanted to get thin, and he put me on a diet. And I stayed on that diet. But I took to it like a religion.

Do you know how truly devout people follow a religion? They learn and observe all the rituals, and they make sure that the religion affects everything about their lives. That is what I did with starvation. Religion is based on belief, and acted out, in part, through rituals. People pray to God for life, happiness, health, money—everything they want or need. Well, I had absolute faith that I would get everything I wanted and needed if I could be thin. And I developed rituals and beliefs to make sure I would get there.

The rituals were really intense, too. I had to prepare my food in only one particular way. I had to then eat only a very specific amount of food. No more, and no less. Like, if we were out to dinner, and you wanted a bite of my chicken, I would let you know in no uncertain terms, don't you dare even ask for a taste of my chicken! I needed exactly the amount I had in mind.

As you might expect, I started to really shed pounds, and everyone around me told me how impressed they were with my willpower. The more I lost, the more elaborate the rituals, and the more overwhelming the praise. I kept lists of good foods...bad foods...foods I could have in the morning, foods I could have at night...everything began to revolve around food. Food, and the scale.

That was when I started weighing myself constantly. Twenty times a day. Just like some people pray to God, I looked to the scale. The scale told me if I was good or evil. You see? Just like a religion.

According to Karen's plan, becoming thin would give her the freedom to be loved and accepted without having to work so hard to please everyone. She always felt that her family and friends responded to her because of what she could do for them, and she was suspicious of them. She suspected that they made fun of her because she was overweight, and she doubted their sincerity in everything they did.

As Karen began to become increasingly involved in losing weight, she was watching to see how family and friends would react to the weight loss. However, since she had never really had a trusting relationship with anyone, she continued to find evidence that the people who said they loved her were really only interested in her because now she was changing. As you will see, some people close to her liked the change very much, but Karen's own feelings were mixed.

* * *

I wish you could have actually seen the different changes going on with different people—all because I was losing weight. What a weird feeling, to know that I was right all along—that these people were more interested in what I weighed than in who I was. Actually, the truth is that I was what I weighed. There was no difference between the number on the scale and the substance of my identity. Think about that. It was bizarre. And everyone in my family was reacting a little bit differently, because I was going through a number of different changes, all related to the weight loss.

The change in my weight really impressed my mother. My father was impressed, too, but my mother was overjoyed. She bragged to all her friends and held me up as an example to all the other fat people she knew, treating me like a real American hero.

It was like she was saying, "See, everybody? This girl was a blimp! And she pulled herself up by her bootstraps, even when she couldn't even see her own bootstraps, and now she's a real person!"

But things between me and my husband were not good. We had a lot of growing-up problems, and I could not have a conversation with him, because he never seemed to listen to what I had to say. Even when I was getting skinny! I couldn't believe it!

So I decided to concentrate my energy where my efforts were being rewarded. And that was in the fatness area. My diet was really the only aspect of my life that was under my control, and so—it took on characteristics that are difficult to explain to someone who hasn't been through it.

You see, as I focused less and less on my husband and everyone else in my family, I developed an intense, personal relationship with my body and with food. I became absolutely obsessed with food. And, because I had no view of anything else, I lost sight of everything else. My food and my body became my security and my belief, just like any love relationship or religion. But it was more than love, or security, or even faith. It was a multilevel relationship between myself and my body. I loved it, hated it—experienced everything I would experience with another person. That's what I had with myself.

You can probably imagine my husband was having a tough time fitting into all of this. But he had ceased to exist for me. So our marriage was over, for all intents and purposes, long before it actually ended. Not that it would have survived, anyway. But I was not involved with him anymore. I was involved with myself. Totally.

I never anticipated this whole withdrawal into myself, and I never really anticipated the pain and unhappiness that would come from not eating. There is just one word to describe how it felt to skip meals and pretend to have eaten. I felt DEPRIVED. DEPRIVED AND CONSTANTLY, PAINFULLY HUNGRY.

I felt completely deprived. You see, I really like to eat. I still like to eat. And I felt, deep in my heart, that something was being taken away from me. And I was angry as hell. I didn't like not eating.

But I did like the things I was getting for not eating. Like the respect that skinny people get. There definitely were good things coming from the starving that I was going through. First of all, I felt more confident. I didn't have to be so friendly and smart and nice, like I did when I was fat. I didn't have to work so hard. In fact, I was allowed to get annoyed, irritable, cranky—all because I was skinny. I started exercising freedom for the first time in my life. And it was delicious!

Not that I liked any of those people around me any more than I did when I was fat. In fact, I liked them less. Because I had contempt for them. Because I felt like I was fooling everyone. And I was! I knew I was the same fat Karen on the inside. But suddenly, all these people, who had always claimed they loved me just for being me, were treating me a whole different way. Like they really did love me, for a change. That stinking, condescending, superior look and tone were GONE.

All my life, I wanted people to see me for me. Not for being fat. And not for being skinny. I was totally convinced that my entire world would change if I could just make myself skinny enough. Then I could go about accomplishing things like everyone else, and they would notice and praise me without prefacing everything by saying, "Wow, even though she's fat, she did that...."

Well, they sure did change. And all I had to do was get skinny. Their perception of me changed. And their reception of me changed. But there was one sickening problem I never thought would come up. MY PERCEPTION OF THEM DIDN'T IMPROVE. In fact, I hated them. No, I resented them more than anything else. Because they were treating me differently. Like a real person, not a fat person. But I was still a fat person.

Right now. This minute. I still think of myself as fat. Even though you and I can see plain as day that I'm skinny. But I'm still a fat girl. Inside.

You know how all these weight-loss programs try to encourage you to stay on a diet because you have a thin person inside, dying to get out? Well, I know I'm a thin person. I can see that I'm thin. But I also know that there is a fat woman inside me, dying to get out. And if she gets out, I'm still afraid that she'll kill me.

I hope I'm expressing myself properly here, because this is important. You have to understand. I don't see my whole body as fat. When I look in the mirror, I don't really see a fat person there. I see certain things about me that are really thin. Like my arms and legs. But I can tell the minute I eat certain things that my stomach blows up like a pig's. I know it gets distended. And it's disgusting. That's what I keep to myself—hug to myself.

Like many people who become anorexic, Karen does not struggle with the idea that she is actually, physically fat. She does fear fat, just the way you may fear snakes, or heights, or a threatening person. She associates fat with death, and it literally scares her to death. So when she consumes even a small amount of food or fluid, her thin and tightly stretched stomach can get distended, and that makes her panic. If you are not anorexic, but you have overeaten at some time in your life, then you know how your stomach can become distended, and you may have to loosen your belt, unbutton your skirt, or adjust your pants for the temporary swelling. While you may experience that swelling after a large meal, Karen's stomach is unaccustomed to holding even the smallest amount of food. Her stomach is somewhat concave—it curves in between her hip bones, and whenever she eats even a small meal, she can feel her stomach become somewhat distended. That distended stomach makes her feel bloated and fat, and she is still as fearful of fat as you might be fearful of death.

I was totally involved with the weight loss, but I was taking the time and effort to notice how people were really behaving toward me, and toward weight issues in general. Ever since I started really losing weight, I've noticed that there are these people out there who say they love me. Or say I'm so thin, wow, how do I keep myself so thin...they say I'm really attractive like this. But I'm the only one who knows what I really am.

You see, I'm really fooling everyone. Because I'm no different inside. I just physically hurt more, because I'm always so hungry. But those people are treating me differently because I'm skinny. That makes me feel really separate from the balance of the world, because the world reacts to the thin me, when I know that the outside Karen has nothing to do with the inside Karen. And I'm thinking to myself, "Ha, ha. You don't know what I'm really like. I have an ugly, horrible secret, and it's more ugly and horrible than all that fat I lost." But it's comfortable. And I keep it a secret. Because it's all that I've got.

You see, for me, the secret is what I hold over the other

people. Every anorexic person is different, but for me, the secret is the obsession. And the obsession is food. Preparing it, attacking it, avoiding it, disposing of it, depriving myself of it, and indulging in it. My obsession. It was all I thought about for EIGHT years.

Everything in my life has to do with food. One way or the other. After a while I start thinking, I have to be very careful. I can't eat even one bite of bread. I can't even put a piece of bread in my mouth. Because the next day, I could wake up fat. I know that other people can put bread in their mouths and they don't wake up fat the next day. But I felt, and still feel, like I just can't afford to take the risk. Like an alcoholic. One swallow would send me straight back to hell.

Can you imagine how much energy it takes to keep up with that kind of demand on your body and your mind? I had no view of anything else. For eight long years, I lost sight of everything but food and my body and my scale and my pain.

That's right. The pain is constant, and intense. And it's always there. So it feels good. Because it's the one thing I can count on. That's the secret for me. It's different for some other people who share my obsession with food and fat. Everyone with my eating problem is different. But that's the way it is for me. The pain is always there. It will never disappoint, the way people disappoint. But there comes a time when you just run out of tricks you can play on your body, and you then start thinking about getting some help. Because everything hurts so much you start to wonder if you're really in control anymore.

It's all such a vicious cycle. You try to take control over your life by really losing weight, and then you find that your weight loss is out of control, and you can't control what your body is doing in response to what you are or are not eating. I started to get the feeling that I could not control the people outside, and I could not control my own body. And if I was that out of control, I could either commit suicide, or go get help. That's when I started to think about going to a doctor.

Naturally, I didn't just wake up one day and look for a doctor. It happened in stages. But the first real reason I went for help was because I was weary of being sick. I was afraid to let go, though. Because, you've got to remember, if I gave it up, I would have nothing. So, I was weary. But I was tremendously afraid. You see, being this skinny is just the flip side of being fat. Just like I got tired of the pressure to be better because I was fat, I started to get tired of being sick.

Sometimes, the actual physical pain would get so intense that I would scream to myself, "I can't go on like this anymore!" But then I would wake up the next day, and there I was—living proof that I could keep going on like that. Because I still was there, right?

Some people say that the worst thing that can happen to you is for your dreams to come true. I guess it depends on what you dream. Because my dream to be totally skinny came true. The only problem was that I remained the same. Inside. In the secret place.

See, I always felt that I could do anything if I were only skinny. Being fat was my excuse for everything I failed at, everything I could not do, and everything I avoided about growing up.

Just as I started thinking maybe I was going to have to face it—that my obsession was not enough—that the big fat excuse was just that—a big, fat excuse, I started noticing a very dangerous pattern. I was gaining weight.

I can remember standing on the scale, my heart pounding, and going over every detail of what I ate, what I drank, how much I exercised—every single minute of every day. Poring over what I had done, trying to find out where I was going wrong. I was sticking to my diet. I really was. But I was still slowly gaining weight.

I knew that if I started with just a little weight, I would go totally out of control. I had visions of blowing up to 300 pounds. After all, I weighed 200 pounds once...maybe I would weigh 300 the next time around. I have to tell you, I got physically ill at the thought. And that's when I decided. If someone could help me eat regularly and still stay thin, then I could be happy. Because I could eat more normally and still find a way to stay thin, with professional help.

So I went to therapists. Psychologists. Social workers. A psychiatrist. And I discovered something very fast. None of them wanted to talk with ME, NOW. They wanted to talk about my childhood, my mother, how I was angry at her or disappointed in my husband. Well, they were right. I did have all those feelings. And I was into a whole self-pitying "I'll-get-you-because-you-made-me-uptight-about-fat" trip. But I was there mainly to take control over the eating, so I could manage the weight. And they just didn't talk with me about *me*. They only talked with me about how I felt about other people.

Look. Let me say this about some of these head doctors. You go to them, literally putting your life in their hands. You're asking them, "What do I do to take back my life? Tell me what to do." And they answered me. I can't say they didn't answer me. But their answers! My God!

They all said more or less the same thing. Like "Try eating a little bit at a time." Can you imagine telling that to me? An anorexic? Someone so totally obsessed with food that no one in the world could have more "eat-a-little-bit-at-a-time" rituals. I mean, I could cut one stalk of asparagus into 21 individual pieces. You just can't eat smaller portions than that. Believe me. I've tried. What else did they say? Things like, "Don't worry about gaining a little weight. People will still find you attractive. You have plenty of room for a few extra pounds." A FEW EXTRA POUNDS! First of all, they were telling me not to worry about getting heavy. You heard that in their words, right? I was a full 30 pounds below the weight I should have been. Good God, I weighed 86 pounds! And they were telling me not to worry about gaining a LITTLE weight. When my entire world revolved around avoiding *any* weight gain. So much so that I went to a doctor to find out why I was beginning to gain—so much so that I didn't know or care about anything else in the world.

I was talking with them. But you can bet they weren't hearing me. So, at the end, I felt that I had deceived absolutely everyone. Even these people, who were supposed to be the experts, believed that my total obsession would just disappear if I would only eat a little. Or if I dated someone, had a sexual relationship, got out of the house more....Look, they were dealing with symptoms. All the symptoms except my obsession.

I really believe they had no idea that I had a serious disorder that made it virtually impossible for me to just blow-dry my hair, put on a new dress, and have dinner in a romantic restaurant, like I was some kind of reluctant recluse who just needed their permission to get out of my little world. I was sick. And weary. And they had no idea at all.

There I was again! The world on one side of reality, and me on the other. As usual, I was standing apart, far away from people who were supposed to know how to help me. But I kept trying, on and off. Because I felt in my soul that if I did not find the right someone to help me, I would die.

That's why I persisted. Because, even when you get this close to pain, this deep inside your own relationship with yourself, you sometimes experience a glimmer of insight into the fact that you can't stay inside yourself forever.

When you have that moment of insight, you know that you really do need a person nearby. Someone who will say, "YOU WANT THE PAIN? HAVE IT. BUT TRY ME. IF YOU WANT TO." It's a long, hard road to move out of that dark side of the soul, where pain is comfort and denial confirms that you're still alive. And I still haven't come out of that world completely. Sometimes, I forget that I can break free. And I doubt.

More and more, though, I believe. I'm replacing my faith in

thinness with faith in myself. And that's exciting. When I think about that, I feel these incredible spurts of joy and confidence. The joy is great, and some of it comes from other people who let me know that there's life out there. And that can take me a long way to confidence.

The treatment for anorexia isn't full of major self-revelations. You don't just wake up one day, decide "to hell with all this" and eat a plate of spaghetti. The treatment takes time. And the insights are small. They come piece by piece. I consciously collect those pieces and assemble them different ways, because I'm trying to make those pieces fit together into a picture. Sometimes, the picture can appear full of promise. But it moves in and out of focus. And I still tend to live on the dark side.

I tend to live there because the pain is comfortable. Like an old sweater that's sort of scratchy. Or the regular route home, even if there's a ton of traffic on that route. Because everything else feels so foreign.

I'm really glad I went for treatment, because I'm beginning to like being alive again...just a little. Actually, I'm really curious about what life can actually offer me. Correct that. I'm a little bit curious. About what I can offer the world, and about what the world can offer me.

Understand this, though. I still don't want to do it alone. I want to explore—and satisfy—small facets of the world outside. But I do not want to explore alone. That's why it's good to be in treatment through this whole healing process.

Basically, I'm at the stage where I'm talking about some of the really gratifying things there are for me in the world. I'm not actually exploring yet. I'm not so sure that I can test the reality outside my secret world, without giving up my obsession with food. But I'm thinking about giving up the obsession, for the first time since all this began. Dropping the religion, so to speak.

You see, I've reached a sort of milestone in therapy, because I can feel that I don't *want* to need the secret and the pain anymore. I can see that my religious focus on food is an obstacle to what I want, instead of an avenue to get what I want. And that is a very big step. But there's still an obstacle I can't get past—yet.

There's just one more thing I want to add. It's something I've been wanting to say all my life. And every single word is important. When a person is fat, don't EVER tell them that they could lose weight if they wanted to badly enough. There was never a time in my life that I wanted it more desperately than any other time. Fat or thin; child, teenager, or adult; single, married, or divorced.

And one more thing. My whole life, I had a fantasy of being thin. I would say to myself, "When I'm thin, I'm coming back to this lousy town and really show these people what I'm made of. I'll break hearts and impress everyone and no one will be able to hurt me again. When I'm thin."

Then I got thin. And I discovered that I had built my whole life around a myth. None of it was true. Not a single word. So now, I'm slowly building on firmer ground.

I'm still in pain. And I'm still tired. But now I have someone beside me that I trust. So, get back to me in a year. Because I'm on my way.

Karen can be proud of how hard she worked to find help. And how hard she continues to work at healing. In fact, she's working on healing with the same singleness of purpose that characterized her intense commitment to losing weight. Can you see how her obsession developed? How she believed, and still believes, that being as skinny as is humanly possible is a guaranteed route to being special?

So far as Karen could tell, everything she did in her entire life was judged and measured in view of the fact that she was fat. If she failed at something, it was because she was fat. And if she succeeded at something, it was a big surprise, because she was fat. She felt that her friends and her family failed to look past her weight to see who she was becoming or how she was getting there.

Karen could never simply enjoy having a date. She felt that she was "the fat girl" who was lucky to find someone willing to give up time to spend with her. And she could never simply get good grades, as far as she was concerned. She had to be at the very top of her class academically, because she felt that she had to be smart to make up for being ugly. And she felt ugly because she had concluded that ugly and fat were the same thing.

Karen felt ugly inside and out. Her memories identify her as a bystander in her own life, incidental to anything good and responsible for everything that went wrong. Skinny or heavy, Karen's experience taught her that her weight was synonymous with her identity to the world and to herself. And her total identity as an overweight person was a deficit. It always meant that she was never good enough.

We can easily identify the steps Karen took toward anorexia. First, she got permission. That permission came from her earliest experiences in school, at home, and on the playground. And you also have to include the permission she got in every message she received from the shows on television, the diet books that lined her walls, and the fitness magazines she subscribed to. All those sources vigorously demonstrated how fat was out, thin was in, and how everyone who was thin looked happy and loved.

Next, Karen developed a set of rituals to manage food. So, in addition to getting permission, she began to obsess about how she prepared food, how much she ate, when she ate, with whom she ate, and how much everyone else ate. She became a gourmet cook, causing her husband to gain 15 pounds very rapidly in the short period before their marriage dissolved. No matter what else happened to her, she knew she could concentrate on food and feel in absolute control over herself and others.

Throughout this process, she worked desperately to keep her secret hidden. After all, people could think she was a freak for actually starving. And people might laugh, since there were many others who managed to lose weight without having to starve. So she would pretend to eat, pretend to go out places, pretend she was part of things. And she kept on losing weight.

In the beginning, everyone around her gave her approval for that effort. But she was the only one who understood what she was really doing, so it became natural for her to retreat inside herself. Because inside herself, she could be who she was. In that way, she began to develop that personal, profound, and exclusive relationship with herself. She began to seek in herself the comfort, support, and response she might ordinarily have sought in another person. She was her only friend, ally, confidante. The only one who knew the truth.

And as she developed that relationship with herself, she began to distrust everyone else. After all, all the people she knew had proved themselves to be unworthy of her trust. Weren't they showing her so much affection since she had lost weight? It was as if they had decided she was a different person. Only she knew that she remained very much the same. In fact, she felt she had gotten much worse, because she was holding close a secret that she called disgusting and ugly.

Without trust in anyone else, she retreated further into herself, focusing exclusively on food. She became convinced that she could get fat overnight. And as she told herself this message over and over again, she developed a deep fear of fat. Fat was the barrier between her and the love she wanted. So fat was always just one morsel away. She felt she could not afford even one bite, unless she militantly apportioned the food. She genuinely distrusted food, because it could turn into fat instantly, so far as she could see.

It's clear how Karen dropped to 30 pounds below a healthy body weight for her age and frame. She learned to fear fat, as you might fear some other danger. And she learned that she was only safe when she was inside herself. Her food rituals and self-involvement filled her day, replacing any people in her life. In a world crowded with friends and family, she was totally isolated.

But staying isolated was hard work. In fact, she found that it was just as exhausting as her efforts to please everyone when she was overweight. Finally, she became tired—sufficiently tired to look for help. And tired enough to keep looking even when she got discouraged. Now she has hope.

Karen is thinking about testing the world again, to see if doors will open to her outside her own world. She says she knows that one door has opened already: the door to treatment. Now that she has that one positive frame of reference, she can open another. At her own pace, in her own time. So she can feel safe enough to let go of the obsession.

Maybe Karen is your daughter. Or she could be your student, friend, patient, wife, or sister. She's right beside you. And now you know that if you keep the door open, she might walk through it today. If she's ready. And if you are ready to make a distinction between what she does, what she weighs, and who she is.

But it might be difficult for you to figure out how to open the door. And it may be even harder to keep it open indefinitely. Sometimes you need some help to keep that door open, and help is available. Asking for it can be difficult, but the reward can be life itself.

5 | The Picture of Health: Jeanette's Story

Beauty, talent, a loving family, wealth, and opportunity. At twelve years old, Jeanette seemed to have everything. Her father, Berton, had earned a reputation as one of the world's leading industrial engineers, consulting with nations and private corporations throughout the world. Her mother, Sarah, remains one of New York's most active patrons of the arts and has a long history of devoting time, effort, talent, and personal funds to support many worthy causes. Then there is Margaret, who is five years older than her sister Jeanette, and is now in college, struggling to make her own way after having had to cope with the fact that her own needs were virtually eclipsed by Jeanette's long withdrawal into anorexia. For Sarah, Jeanette's mother, the collective and individual suffering the family has endured is far from over. But it has reached a positive turning point.

Every family shares moments that are especially close and lovely. Our family enjoyed such a time during the summer that Jeanette turned twelve. For the first time in over a decade, our entire family had a grand reunion at our home in

Southampton. Everyone on both sides of the family came—from Connecticut, Georgia, Wisconsin, upstate New York—everywhere. The festivities lasted for days, but the reunion itself took place on one of those magical summer days—warm and dry and absolutely perfect.

I wish I could show you the photographs. They're perfect. Everyone was radiant, and the pictures captured that spirit. It was just a happy day, everyone getting involved in all kinds of games, and Jeanette stood out in the crowd, the picture of health, with that exquisite tan she gets, and a wonderful mane of auburn hair that positively gleams in the sun. It is still impossible for me to imagine that it would be just four months before it would be clear to anyone who looked that my beautiful, glowing child was dangerously ill.

But before I get to that, you need to have a little background. You see, Jeanette was always very beautiful. From the day she was born, everyone always said she was the most adorable little girl. As a matter of fact, she was a model for baby products when she was still an infant, and her looks never disappeared. You know how some children can be very beautiful for a short period of time? Well, Jeanette never had an awkward phase. She just became prettier as time went by.

I must say I have always been proud of that. It really didn't matter that she was always a little chubby. It was part of her total self, her special beauty. And she wasn't just pretty. She was talented. She has very definite musical ability and is quite an accomplished pianist now. She was already clearly talented while she was still in elementary school, and she has had many opportunities to perfect and perform her art.

When it came to day-to-day schoolwork, Jeanette exerted herself the same way she did when she practiced piano. She gave every bit of herself to the effort. She has always been a perfectionist that way, but she never seemed to get any satisfaction from what she produced. It was simply never enough for her. No matter how well she excelled, no matter how much praise she received, it was never enough.

You could praise her around the clock. It didn't matter. It never got through. That was always the frustration. You could admire her and explain to her how or why her work was admirable, and she would dismiss everything you said. She never seemed to know how to absorb the wonderful things.

But I'm getting ahead of myself again. You see, these were always features of Jeanette's personality, and I have to tell you, I felt she would naturally outgrow those problems as she developed confidence. I thought she would develop confidence by building up a history of successes, which she was doing. It seemed to me that she had the usual needs and imperatives, and that anything else would just work itself out over time. She got so much praise from us, from her teachers, from her friends...how could she do anything but grow out of that childhood tendency to diminish her accomplishments or her beauty?

So, when you ask what the first signs of her illness were, I suppose some of those signs were in place for much of her life. But the first severe, physical signs developed shortly after Jeanette entered junior high school. You see, she took on the challenge of junior high with great spirit. She was very happy to start a new life, in a new building, with all new teachers, and she resolved to go back to school in September "looking different." You can see some of that difference in the photographs I was telling you about, from the reunion. That reunion took place in the summer before Jeanette entered seventh grade, and she had already begun to lose weight.

I remember her announcing to us all that there would be no more adorable, chubby-little-girl image for her! She didn't want to be known as the cuddly little girl who tried the hardest. She wanted a reputation as the slender, successful young woman who would command everyone's attention and respect.

I must admit I was happy about the whole thing. So was Berton. We were happy that she wanted to continue to improve her image. And we were happy when she wanted to lose weight. In fact, before she launched her self-improvement program, I had been thinking of talking to her pediatrician about putting her on a diet, because she is big-boned, and she was putting on weight—a little more each year. She loved food so much, and she always had a sweet tooth. I never allowed junk food in the house, but she would buy it somehow on her own, and hoard it. I knew what she was doing, and I was concerned that the slight chubbiness would become a problem as she got older.

As it turned out, I never had to bring it up with the pediatrician. Jeanette decided to lose weight just before school started. When she started seventh grade, Jeanette was about five feet, two inches tall, and weighed 110 pounds. But the time she went for her general checkup in October, she was down to 98 pounds. That means she lost 12 pounds in four weeks.

From all outside appearances, she had set a goal for herself, and she was achieving it. I was concerned that she had lost the weight that fast, but I decided to be cool about it. I knew my daughter. She was going through a difficult time of adjustment, and I felt she would get angry and just give up completely if I said that she was losing weight the wrong way. I genuinely believed that she needed to know she was excellent at this whole diet and self-image change. It was part of being noticed in a positive way, and I wanted to reinforce what I saw as a healthy direction she was taking. After all, she had a goal, and was working hard to achieve it. That had to be good.

It's important that you understand I did not decide that course of action on my own. I asked the pediatrician how we should respond to that weight loss. And he told me in no uncertain terms. He had actually planned to put Jeanette on a diet that October, because he was also concerned about her weight, now that she was entering adolescence. Particularly since she had always been inclined to overeat, especially junk food. So. The doctor said it, and Berton and I agreed. I remember thinking, "Oh! This is wonderful! This child is taking charge of her life! Being very discriminating! Choosing what she wants and when she wants it, all with so much control! This is what growing up is all about!"

Now I know that she was experiencing a precipitous drop in weight, and that sharp decline was a warning. The first physical sign of trouble. But the doctor didn't say there was any cause for concern, and I had no reason to believe anything was wrong. I was a little in shock, but I was happy. You have to realize, she was not petite at 98 pounds. She wasn't even thin. Her frame is large, and at that point she gave the appearance of looking very healthy. No one suspected that she was ill. Not even her pediatrician.

Jeanette was clearly determined to change the way her life was going. She was frustrated with her school performance and hated herself for having difficulty with food, especially since it seemed to her that her mother had everything together, from head to toe. It did not occur to Jeanette that her mother had been through her own stressful and disappointing times. In fact, it was impossible for Jeanette to imagine that her mother was anything less than perfect. Jeanette was desperate for something that would make her special—admired and respected for something she created herself, through her own initiative.

Sarah admired and understood that need but never had a clue that such a normal human need could manifest itself in such a profoundly self-destructive way. As a parent, Sarah was proud that her daughter could develop such strong goal orientation, especially toward controlling an aspect of personal health and nutrition that was so important to Sarah. Her daughter had a chance to start over again, in a new school, with the potential to make new friends and achieve new accomplishments—including control over her own health and eating habits. On the surface, it was a scenario any parent would celebrate, especially when the youngster is a teenager.

The teen years are as confusing for adults as they are for

teenagers themselves. It can be very difficult to figure out what is and is not okay in adolescent behavior. Now, Sarah knows that a parent who is confused should keep looking for professional guidance and input until she, or he, finds satisfactory support. Today, Sarah understands that the entire family, plus teachers and the pediatrician, all lavishly praised Jeanette for her weight loss. From Jeanette's point of view, that lavish praise was equivalent to permission to go as far as humanly possible in getting thin. No one thought to ask her how she felt about it, or whether she had mixed feelings. No one thought to ask how she thought her life would change if she lost weight, and no one even considered the possibility that Jeanette's goal weight might be unhealthy. After all, everything she was doing appeared to be health oriented.

When things began to get out of hand, there were clear signs. Sarah freely admits that the signs of some disturbance were evident fairly early. She just had no idea what to do, or whether the whole thing would pass, like some sort of growing pain. So she waited and tried to ignore that her daughter was rapidly becoming a stranger.

At first, everyone was really impressed with Jeanette's progress. She was so focused, it was incredible. She had seen the doctor during the second week of October, in the first semester of seventh grade, just two months after the family reunion. It was early in November that the first clear signs showed that something just wasn't right. All of a sudden, there were very few things that were acceptable to her. She had decided to become a vegetarian, like her sister, and I didn't think that was so bad. It was a good diet. But it was a very glum period. She had begun to look so depressed, and she clearly had lost the energy that always vitalized her—always shone from inside, that made her especially lovely. You could see the change in her skin, the look in her eyes, and especially in the way she walked.

And her clothes! I know teenagers go through stages

where they express rebellion through clothes. I understood that then, and expected it as a stage. But all she wore was pants and a sweatshirt. The same black pants, skin tight, and the same black sweatshirt. Day in. And day out. She would wash her clothes so they would be clean, but they were always the same.

At that point, even her friends seemed to think she was dressing and behaving in an extreme way. I recall that one of the older girls in school told her mother that she thought we, Jeanette's parents, should do something. I bumped into her mother when I was food shopping one day, and she mentioned that comment to me. She seemed somewhat embarrassed, and she explained that her daughter was so troubled, she felt it was only right to convey those concerns to me.

What was I to do? Of course, I thanked her. Thanked her warmly. I knew she was right. We all knew she was right. But we were so afraid of talking about it at home. Or anywhere else. We still felt it was a phase, something that would pass if ignored.

So no one said anything at home. Berton and I resolved that part of it could be that we all were drifting away from each other—between his work, my activities, and each daughter growing up so fast and choosing different ways to fill every day. Berton and I discussed this whole matter of how we were all going very fast in different directions, and we decided that we could help the whole thing if we went on a family trip. A really grand vacation to France, for the Christmas holiday. All of us together, doing the same thing.

We have pictures of that trip. The black-and-whites definitely say more. She looked so dismal, and the pictures are so poignant. They are the first pictures of her when she was clearly desperately ill. And we were still silent, struggling to keep the family together, going through the motions of doing everything any other family would do on a vacation to France.

We went to all the museums, went on walking tours of gardens and villages, and shopped like mad. Naturally, we went to the restaurants in all the different quarters, to try the various specialties, and every day would start out the same way. We would have breakfast, which she would not eat. At lunch, she would relent enough to swallow some consommé, a little plain bread, or maybe a salad. That's all she would eat, and she was very grudging about it.

Dinner was out of the question. She would repeat her breakfast performance. So it got to the point where we would eat our main meal at lunch and would avoid a family meal in the evening. All in all, throughout the entire trip, at every stop and every museum, our entire focus was on her. I think I could go back now and find almost nothing familiar. We were all watching her so intently, the whole landscape had rapidly become incidental.

My other daughter, Margaret, would catch us when we were all walking. Jeanette would walk so far ahead of us, especially after lunch—always working off calories, ready to walk another mile, and Margaret would take that opportunity to talk with us. About how Jeanette frightened her, she was so thin. She was sharing a room with her sister, while Berton and I had our own room, of course. And Margaret was able to see her sister dress every day. Every day, she would put on the same black pants, the same loose black shirt, and the same wide, black belt. She wrenched that belt around her waist so tightly it frightened Margaret. Naturally, Margaret was worried about her sister, so she would whisper to us that Jeanette's belt was so tight that it was rubbing off her skin...God. We all felt so helpless and confused.

But that belt was Jeanette's control, and she was determined to wear it as tightly as possible. It told her she was right, that she was losing weight, and it told her when she had eaten enough. As soon as she felt additional pressure on that belt she would immediately stop eating. Maybe that sounds like a good idea—to wear a belt that reminds you that you've had enough. Well, she still has scars on her abdomen from that belt.

You can't imagine how it was at meals. Lunch was the only meal we all would really focus on, because the food was so rich, and we wanted to enjoy it. We didn't want to overeat at dinner and then go directly to sleep. Even if we did want to indulge on a given day, Jeanette would never participate, so we all avoided such dinner scenes. That meant that our main meal was lunch, but I cannot remember the details of any food, the tension was so great. I know that Berton and I drank a lot of wine at lunch every day. It helped get us through her obsessive behavior, which I have to explain for you, because it's crucial that you visualize and feel just what she was like during this period.

For instance, there was the way she would eat her food. How she would separate each bit of food, cut it into tiny, precise shapes, and repeatedly calculate calories on a small counter that clicked. She had that calorie system down to a science, and she would continually pore over what she had on her plate, what she could eat, and how much or how little she might gain. My God, it could take her an hour just to prepare the food that was served to her on her plate—cutting, shaping, dividing. . . . Lunch could be interminable. Imagine yourself thinking about having to go through such a meal, and then sitting through it, wishing it were over, but desperately hopeful that some new sort of behavior would develop—something that would show that your beautiful young girl wanted to live a normal life.

By the end of the trip, she had lost another ten pounds and had broken the belt one day when she tried harder than usual to tighten it. Our holiday had been an exercise in futility, and Berton and I knew we had to go for help. In fact, we all agreed, including Margaret. Jeanette was so gaunt, she was disappearing in front of our eyes. But she wanted to go to a doctor because, she said, her stomach hurt her often.

* * *

Sarah, Berton, and Jeanette went through a very typical process before they accepted the fact that they genuinely needed help. First, Sarah and Berton gave their daughter clear permission to lose weight, never anticipating that such an ordinary goal could raise such crucial issues of personal control and closely held feelings of guilt, self-hatred, anger, and frustration.

Basically, they followed the ordinary health and education planning for their daughter, relying on the professionals at school and in the medical profession to tell them if something was right, or wrong, with their daughter. There is no record that anyone said that anything seemed to be wrong, and there are several records testifying to the fact that the pediatrician involved also gave Jeanette permission to lose weight without discussing with her the other, more elusive goals she expected to achieve in the process. No one anticipated that this apparently happy, pretty girl with every advantage in the world could possibly be suffering such intensely conflicting and self-destructive feelings.

As Jeanette's behavior began to deteriorate, it was tempting to attribute the change to adolescence. Both Sarah and Berton believed that, as parents, they were supposed to understand their daughter well enough to know that this deterioration was just a phase. They did not even think of asking a medical doctor, psychologist, or social worker if this was normal behavior for a teenager. They simply believed that they would know if it was serious, because they were good parents. So they put enormous pressure on themselves to diagnose their daughter's elusive needs, and Jeanette put equal pressure on herself to reach the very limits of her tolerance for pain on her way to reaching the all-important goal to become as thin as possible.

As Jeanette and her parents became increasingly isolated in their own concerns and frustrations, they began to share one common interest: the need for professional guidance and support. Jeanette actually wanted advice because it was getting impossible for her to lose weight, no matter what she did. In fact, she was beginning to gain a few ounces every day, and she was virtually in a state of panic.

Sarah and Berton agreed that it was important to go for help, because they could see that ignoring the problem, or waiting for it to pass, were unsuccessful coping strategies. So, with Jeanette's active support, Sarah began to look for professional help.

When there is ill health in the family, you're willing to try anything. Travel. Special strategies. Costly treatment. Anything. Just to find the right kind of help. I can tell you, I was desperate. So when we got back from France, the first step I took was to talk with my neighbor, who is a psychiatrist with a very fine reputation. He suggested that I call Mr. Curan, who was a social worker in Brooklyn Heights. He was also a lovely man, very well respected, but I could tell right away that he knew too little. He was advising her to put on a few pounds, not to worry so much, not to be so anxious about school work—he was trying to soothe her, but she was beyond that.

Once we all agreed that we had to find some help, I started a search that became as bizarre and exhausting as one of those complicated movie plots that you think never could happen in real life. First, I called two psychologists in Manhattan, and they both took several days to get back to me. I waited and waited, and they did call back, just to tell me that they were too busy to accept new patients. One of my friends told me a nutritionist might help, that she had heard of a nutritionist who had experienced some success with young women who refused to eat. So I took Jeanette to that particular nutritionist, and I said to myself, "Even if he is a semi-quack, I have to try. I have to try everything."

He said that she had to start taking vitamins, that something showed up in her nail clippings. She was convinced that the vitamins were full of calories, and she never really took them. In the meantime, while we have been running around looking for help, Jeanette's schoolwork was suffering, and she was showing no physical signs of healing.

It's difficult for me to explain here how frightened I was. No one was helping, no matter how hard I tried. My husband was worried, and he was very good to me, very supportive, but he had his work, and he had to travel frequently. I knew this was my job, this business of finding help. And I had to succeed. If I didn't, I felt my child might die. So I pulled myself together again, and I called a doctor who is a neighbor of mine in Southampton, and who has been recognized as being an authority in eating disorders like anorexia. At that point, I was convinced that Jeanette had anorexia.

That doctor, who was also a good friend, did call back, of course, and took some of Jeanette's history over the phone. She already knew a great deal, of course, having been my neighbor for fifteen summers. Her son has always been a friend of Jeanette's, and we had all gotten along well over the years. She listened to the whole story very patiently and explained very carefully that she felt the personal aspect of the relationship would be a problem. At any rate, she was not accepting any new patients, because she was overbooked as it was.

She told me all this very gently, but I could feel my entire body getting rigid with fear, rage, anxiety—another dead end! But she did tell me to listen carefully, that she was not abandoning me. She would refer me to a doctor she had heard was having considerable success with patients who were anorexic. That doctor turned out to be Dr. Sacker.

I was shaking when I got off the phone. I don't think I could have stood too many more rejections. I had really used up all my resources, and I was frantic. When Dr. Sacker agreed to see us at Brookdale Hospital in Brooklyn, I was inexpressibly relieved. I knew—I foresaw that this would be a long, difficult ordeal, and it was a comfort that he was so close to home.

All this time, Jeanette knew I was looking for a doctor. There was nothing secret in all this. She and Berton and I had discussed the whole thing a number of times, and she said, "YES, I want to see a doctor." I have to say she was very

open to help. There was no question that she wanted someone to understand and help her. And it was very clear that it
was my job to get that help when we got back from France.
My husband was very sad—sad and concerned and kind of
helpless. His work was so consuming and stressful, he couldn't
be part of searching for the right doctor. But he was always
involved. Through me.

Anyway, Jeanette and I went to the doctor's office, and I
can recall each moment of driving there, meeting the doctor,
sitting in the waiting room....It was, in a word, memorable.
You have to envision this now. There was all the usual hassle
of traffic, parking, the anxiety of being in a hospital....Anyway,
as soon as we entered Dr. Sacker's office, we saw a child who
was much sicker than Jeanette—a gorgeous black girl who I
understand was hospitalized shortly after that day. She was
sitting with her great-aunt, directly across from us, and that
old, elegant lady looked at us very clinically. We were there
maybe half a minute, and that woman said, "She's got the
same problem as mine," and she was looking straight at
Jeanette. It was unnerving, but I was more involved with how
Jeanette would react. And what was going to happen next.

You see, I was anticipating any number of scenarios.
Mostly, I wanted a script. I wanted to know exactly what to do
next. While I was sitting there, waiting for Jeanette to come
out of that doctor's office, I kept wondering, what would I do
if this was the wrong place? Whom else could I call? Was
Jeanette really going to get well? Or would she just continue
to get worse, like that incredibly beautiful black girl who was
sitting across from me, dressed in a chic, layered outfit of all
different, vivid colors, looking like a cover girl except for her
eyes. They were almost opaque.

Anyway, I knew the moment I saw my daughter's face that
this doctor could help. Her face had been completely cheer-
less for more than six weeks, and when my child walked out
of that first session, she was smiling. It was like finding water
in the desert. Let me tell you, he gained my confidence that

day, mostly because of the expression on my daughter's face. She looked as if she had finally discovered someone who really knew what she was going through. You might have the same expression on your face if you were stuck in a foreign country where no one spoke English, and you found someone from your own home town. You would probably feel relieved, excited, safer, happier, and hopeful. Most of all, hopeful—and all those feelings would show on your face. Well, that's how Jeanette looked. And that was my first clue that this was a person who could help.

For me, it also helped that the doctor was an M.D., associated with an established hospital in the community. But it wasn't just the diplomas. It was the instinct I had. I was positive he could help. He exudes compassion, and he is totally straightforward. That way, his style matched her style, and mine. If I was the sort of person who needed a different type of help, maybe I wouldn't have been as happy. But our styles matched, and he seemed to understand her problem. That was all-important. So many doctors and therapists are good at what they do, but they have no idea how to approach this special problem.

He was also very affirmative. He said it would take him some time to see if he could help. So, within two or maybe three sessions, he told me he did believe that he could help her heal. All these things are important things to look for in a professional person. You want them to take time, to think about your special needs. And I liked something else. He gave ME time. Not that he ever violated his promise to Jeanette to keep their sessions private. He never betrayed her confidence. But he did give me extra time, which was very important to me.

I hear about other parents who are totally excluded from therapy for eating disorders and other certain problems, and I wonder how it can work. As a matter of fact, one of my friends was telling me the other day that her daughter has suffered from anorexia for ten years, and that she has never known what was going on in her daughter's treatment. The anorexia is still unresolved, and her daughter is 24 years old now ... still hitting weights like 88 pounds, and the girl is five foot seven.

You see, I was happy that this doctor would listen to me, because I had a lot to say, and I had to have someone I could trust who would listen to me. I didn't want to tell my friends everything. And Berton and I had reached the point where we couldn't talk about it. I needed to get my daughter a doctor who could also listen to me, and reassure me, if there was reassurance to offer.

When Jeanette walked out of that office, she was motivated to get help, and she said so out loud. She said that her bizarre eating habits upset her and were taking a toll on her appearance, which was also getting her nervous. Even though she had developed incredible energy, there were other side effects that were beginning to make her very unhappy. Like what was happening with her hair.

That blonde hair, which had always been so thick and glossy, was getting brittle and falling out in bits and pieces. Even worse, her face, throat, arms, her whole body was getting covered with this strange light hair that made her very self-conscious, and she wanted to get rid of it. All these symptoms were part of her anorexia, and she didn't like these new developments. She seemed to feel this doctor could help her get rid of these problems. So the first visit was really a turning point.

Right from the start, the doctor focused on finding out what Jeanette really wanted in the near future. Well, what she really wanted was to enter a particular race. It was a six-mile race, and she would be competing with adults and other young people. Well, at this point in her life, she was 13 and weighed 79 pounds. He told her that she could train for that race if—and only if—she began to gain some weight. He never said exactly how much weight, and he never got caught up in telling her exactly what to eat. He has never gotten involved in any of her food games, listing foods she can or can't eat, or anything like that.

I can't tell you anything specifically about the treatment that unfolded for her between her and her doctor in the privacy of the sessions. But I can tell you that she responded beautifully, right from the start. She built her weight up, he allowed her to train for running, and she was totally committed to that training. Actually, she reached a reasonable, safe weight just two weeks before that race, and she came in third against a field of runners that included her own father, whom she beat! She actually did a better time than Berton, who is quite an accomplished, seasoned runner himself.

Commitment was the hallmark of this doctor's approach, and it's a quality I would look for in any other doctor who works with people who have anorexia. If Jeanette had a goal, and it involved a physical activity, she had to demonstrate her commitment to that goal by eating a balanced set of meals every day, and by gaining weight. Over the time that her weight was stabilizing, she started to notice that the rest of the world existed, and she developed some new interests that were really very nice.

For instance, she got involved in climbing mountains. She researched the different camps specializing in that sort of challenge and presented the doctor with the idea that climbing would be good for her. Well, he told her that it was too scary for him to let her go just on her word. She had to show her commitment.

She did that. Oh, boy, did she do it! Right on the button. She hit precisely the weight they agreed would be safe, based on the literature about climbing, and she went off to camp with his blessing. She excelled at everything there, won medals for all sorts of things, and came back from that camp convinced that she was a new person. She was superior at everything they had asked her to try, had outdone many older, bigger girls and boys, and had shown great courage and sportsmanship.

When she went back to school that fall, she looked gorgeous. She had been in treatment for just about six months, the camp experience had really boosted her confidence, and she was determined to succeed at everything in school, just as she had succeeded at camp. Like everything else she has ever done in her life, she did this with a passion, with every ounce of energy she had.

Throughout the first four months of school, she got good grades, did her work, made new friends, and gave up old friends who she felt would not fit into this new life of hers. She appeared to be turning into a healthy, well-adjusting eighth grader, and one of the best pieces of news we got was that she weighed 120 pounds. With all that going for her, the doctor felt she was stable enough to go to Europe for Christmas. She said she wanted to go, and the rest of us felt that we really needed and deserved a break. We all felt so good about Jeanette's progress, and we were all certainly due for a good vacation.

It's important for you to understand that even this healing process was exhausting. True, we were finally getting help. But everything was still a struggle. She was always asking if she looked good, always needed assurance about her arms, waist, face, cheekbones, the condition of her hair, and all that fuzz she had grown.... It was so hard to tell what she might find offensive. I did learn very quickly that the worst thing you could say to her was that she was healthy looking, because to look healthy meant to look robust, and robust meant fat, as far as she was concerned. So it was very difficult to be encouraging, because I never really knew how she would feel about what I was saying.

So, I would check with Dr. Sacker. But no one can anticipate everything. She needed so much. She would ask over and over again if she was getting too fat, if she really looked pretty in a particular dress or color.... Sometimes, I was just at my wits' end with all her questions and insecurity.

On top of all that, there was the added and undeniable fact

that she was gaining weight, and it was getting more and more visible. I clearly remembered Dr. Sacker warning that sometimes people can swing from anorexia to obesity—that they stay compulsive and obsessive, and actually reverse the outcome for weight. I was genuinely afraid of that, and I know I had difficulty with that fear. On the one hand, I was afraid that she would die of starvation. On the other hand, I was almost equally fearful that she would destroy herself by becoming obese.

You have to remember, Jeanette did have something of a weight problem throughout her childhood. I know that other people may not have found her heavy, but I could see the tendency in her frame and in her eating habits, and it was always a concern. The doctors agreed, even when she was very young. So she was inclined to weight gain in the first place. Now that inclination was compounded, it seemed, because she had this anorexia, which made her susceptible to rapid, excessive weight gain. She did have to watch her calories, or she would get fat. But how do you ask a girl suffering from anorexia to actually watch her calories?

I was sure that I was losing my mind. I felt like I was living inside a hideous maze, where every choice was a dead end. I was fearful to support her in any health-oriented or eating-behavior goal, because I generally could not determine what was and was not moderate eating behavior for my own child. Can you imagine how anxious that made me, and the rest of my family? We were constantly on edge.

So I was afraid to get into the food thing with her too much. I held back most of the time. Berton and Margaret stayed away from the topic completely. We were all very, very careful, and Jeanette reached the 120-pound level just before the Christmas holiday. As I said, we were all so incredibly stressed—so we decided that a vacation would help. Since it was the holiday season, we consulted with her doctor, and he said it would be safe to go away together and travel anywhere else but where we had been the last time we all went away.

He warned that Jeanette might need to assert control in the old, familiar, destructive way, but that she would probably not lose a dangerous amount of weight. So, prepared with that understanding, we decided that the family would benefit from a vacation together in Italy and Switzerland.

Well, as soon as we were in Italy, she decided to be in control again, just as the doctor said might happen. She lost 10 pounds, and I couldn't help feeling in my heart that I was glad she lost the weight, because she looked beautiful. Every day she made the point that she had lost the 10 pounds because she decided she would. When she would ask us if we thought she looked good, we had to say it was true. She did look lovely. Her clothing was pretty, her hair was getting healthier, and there was no dreadful belt cinched around her waist like a vise.

When we came home again, Dr. Sacker was concerned about the 10-pound weight loss, but he never harped on it. He kept focused on how she could set goals and achieve them, so she could gain control over positive objectives in her life. The first big goal was to get in touch with her feelings about teenage growing-up things, like how she felt about school and how she could learn to cope with boys. All those regular, adolescent issues that Jeanette had never really talked about before.

I suppose you could say that the treatment has evolved slowly from an emphasis on physical strengthening to an emphasis on emotional strengthening. With this treatment plan, my daughter has gained the weight she needs and has stayed on a balanced diet. I know that she eats too many sweets once in a while, but she has come so far! Now she is more and more involved in getting through to her own feelings, which she was very separate from when she was sick.

It seems that Jeanette's weight is stabilized at this point, but I still feel that we are all at risk. She is not out of danger yet. At this point, we can only measure her safety and security by degrees—no absolutes. She is not safe or unsafe. She is okay today, but her position is risky. Right now, she seems to have no real weight-loss problem. She's eating good, solid, balanced meals, and she's even taking a multivitamin, according to doctor's orders. She still says things like, "I know it's silly, Mom, but I just want to make sure...these vitamins don't have too many calories, right?" So she still does keep track of calories, and she does tend to sneak snacks.

Basically, she cooks for herself, totally. There are really two sets of meals being produced in my kitchen: hers and ours. It would actually be something of a relief that she does her own cooking, since she's still fairly particular, but it drives me crazy, because she always leaves such a mess. I know that this is a much less serious problem than anorexia, but I can't always be so thankful that she's alive that I don't allow myself to feel any anger toward her. Her way of getting rid of a pot is to put it away, even if it's dirty. So when I reach for a pot, it's greasy or crusty. I hate it. Most people don't have to put up with that shit.

You see, I feel right now that things are just so much more positive. So I cannot complain about each thing that makes me upset. I have to choose my battles, and the kitchen mess is not one of them. I can't fight it all. I prefer to see the total picture, and the total picture is getting more positive. She has new friends, she looks wonderful, and she has only been sick one day this whole semester, which is very nearly over. Plus, she's taking her vitamins every day, and that's a giant step toward protecting her health. She never took an active role in getting or staying healthy before. On the whole, I can say that she is more safe than she was. And, she seems to improve as far as her weight and physical health are concerned.

The question right now is, what direction will this disorder take now? Where will it go? There is no such thing as just recovering from anorexia and sailing through the rest of your life without incident. Anorexia can be overcome very specifically, in terms of weight gain and eating habits. But it takes longer for the individual and the family to recover...to develop new lines of communication. We all have to learn to stop using food or weight issues to deal with our feelings, and Jeanette is not the only one in the family re-learning how to interact with each other in a healthy way.

As a parent, I ask "What would be the worst thing now? Now that she is physically better?" Sexual promiscuity? So far, that has not been a problem, thank God. In fact, her concern is that there are all these boys, and she just wants to flirt. Nothing else. She really talks to me about this. She asks if she is responsible for everything just because she flirts, and she wants to know who is responsible in every kind of social interaction.

So she's going over all this in therapy. She feels her doctor knows her inside out—everything she's thinking. He's responded to that faith by giving her the messages and confidence she needs to handle all those social pressures. He keeps on delivering the message that her body is her own, and she can decide to protect her body from harm that could be inflicted by herself, or by anyone else. That's a direct appeal to the positive side of her ability to set limits for herself and others.

So the sexual promiscuity has not been an issue. Yet. But there have been other issues. Profoundly unsettling, even heartbreaking. You see, the obsession that manifests itself in that intense weight loss doesn't necessarily go away with weight stabilization. It can go from one thing to the next. The latest thing has been that she has lied over and over again, to the point where it's difficult to determine what is fact, and what is fiction.

Sarah's struggle to understand and anticipate her daughter's behavior has been frustrated by the fact that Jeanette is still learning how to express her feelings in an acceptable way. She spent her entire life developing ways to hold her feelings inside and please everyone important to her. Those efforts to please everyone were made at great cost, because it became increasingly difficult for her to believe that she could do or say how she really felt, unless she thought that her parents and teachers and friends would approve.

When you spend your entire life trying to please other people at the expense of pleasing yourself, then you can become angry. You may find it difficult to express that anger, because that might offend the people you are trying to please. Then you may feel angry at the people you're trying to please, because they make you feel that you have to be perfect.

You may consciously or subconsciously turn that anger onto yourself, because you may feel that hurting yourself is a good way of hurting other people. Anorexia is just one disorder that can develop when you turn your anger inward so that you can hurt others without actually appearing to hurt them.

When you enter into treatment to help understand and overcome the anorexia, you may stabilize your weight and begin to practice some healthy eating, sleeping, and exercise habits. And that is when you reach a new level of risk, because you may begin to express your anger in new ways.

As Jeanette has developed more healthy eating and exercise habits, and her school performance has improved, she has begun to face and cope with all the anger she has always felt in response to the pressure she felt to achieve. While she continues to attempt new and more appropriate ways to express all different types of positive and negative feelings, she may also engage in inappropriate ways of expressing anger. That means she may steal, or lie, or fail in school. Or she may do other things that cause her harm, because her primary and original coping mechanism has been to deny and hide angry feelings, and hurt others by hurting herself.

As Jeanette learns to express feelings in a more appropriate way, her life, like her weight, will become more balanced. That balance will only be achieved over time, and the time it takes can be brutal on the family.

* * *

It's heartbreaking and infuriating to have to face the fact that my daughter lies to me about things—the most ridiculous, minor things . . . and the lies have been compounded by stealing—stealing from us, her family! She's been stealing from my room, her sister's room, and from the house in general. Important things, things that have great sentimental value. Sometimes the things turn up again, but sometimes they don't. And she lies about taking the things.

It has been a terrible assault on my heart, this stealing and lying. I get really hurt. The things she has taken from me were all gifts from my husband—her father. It seems that she's so angry at him. That anger gets expressed in all kinds of direct and indirect ways. Of course he reacts. Sometimes with anger, sometimes with sarcasm. Sometimes he just withdraws in pain.

I know that Jeanette is learning new ways to express and experience anger, disappointment, and even joy. She has stopped starving herself, and she's stopped playing very dangerous food games. Now she needs to address her feelings, and that's frightening for her, and for the rest of us. Because if she had such powerfully dangerous feelings that she could nearly destroy herself, what is she to do with those feelings now? What were they? And how will they be brought out and resolved?

Those questions are slowly being answered in therapy. But in the process, it's unnerving to keep trying to anticipate when and where her anger will surface next. Right now, all that punishing emotion is directed at me and at her father. I understand that all the lying and stealing are just part of that. But it's still difficult, and damn near impossible to take sometimes.

Meanwhile, she's also been having trouble in school. She refuses to do any work that presents a challenge. In fact, the only schoolwork she actually finishes are the assignments that she can do without risking any kind of failure. She's been avoiding projects that were due and are now overdue.

So there's the difficulty with school, and the stealing at

home. Money has been missing from the house, along with clothing and jewelry. I've gotten wrapped up in trying to anticipate the incidents, while I'm trying to sort out what takes place as it develops. I try to be direct and to the point, but how can you be so clear when you're dealing with someone who is so unclear? So, even though she seems safe from the jeopardy that comes from starvation, at least at this moment, there are all these other concerns. There is still the whole cycle of lying and stealing, which obliges me to cut through for the truth. It takes so much energy, and I am very tired. Tired, and sad, and angry. Then, naturally, the question looms, what will happen next?

The trust is really gone, you see. And I've never been in a relationship with anyone where I have lost trust. I would never have expected such a violation of trust with my own daughter. On top of that disappointment, she is just so difficult to deal with. I can remember, early in her treatment, she and Dr. Sacker decided on a weight level that would be the best for her to achieve in order for her to go on a hiking and climbing expedition. She took it right to the ounce. That's when he told me, "You're dealing with a tough young woman. Coping with her is going to demand great stamina on your part." Truer words were never spoken. I just want to know how much more stamina I can expect from myself.

She's always driving home the same message. Over and over, everything she does screams out the message, "Look at me! I am in control! I have more self-control than you! And I can sabotage anything you have that I want or that I want to take away from you!" She does have great willpower. It is true that she can accomplish anything she wants. When she says she will lose 10 pounds, she loses 10 pounds. It can be hard to take, because you can begin to resent her power. If she's so powerful, so capable of action, why does she insist on acting in a way that so clearly hurts herself, and her family? The answer seems to be that she wants to do that damage, and that possibility is hard to accept.

Meanwhile, the family has been dramatically affected. I know now that my older daughter Margaret just gave up on trying to compete with her sister while Jeanette was ill. I don't blame her. How can you share a stage with someone who has anorexia? She wanted to help, so she was no problem to anyone. She simply withdrew and waited until the immediate, life-threatening situation was resolved. In fact, she had always been somewhat underweight, but all that was eclipsed during Jeanette's most difficult period. Now, Margaret is away at college and is about 20 pounds overweight. So it never stops. First one, then the other.

With it all, I cannot forget what Dr. Sacker told me the first time we spoke. He said that more families dissolve over this problem than not. I learned that I had to treat relationships in the family gently, because statistics were not in our favor. A family is alternately fragile and strong, and our family was fragile in some very special ways. In some ways, there is just no end of giving.

Sometimes I say to myself, "I don't think it has to be this hard." And I ask, "Why us?" But I think we feel fairly guilt-free most of the time. I have dear friends, and family, who have even more burdensome troubles, and I remind myself that I must keep this whole problem in some sort of perspective. That's one of the reasons why it's important for me to be able to talk with her doctor sometimes. Not to find out about Jeanette necessarily, but to talk with him about my feelings.

He did explain to me at the beginning that he was Jeanette's doctor, and that I should feel free to enter into therapy on a regular basis with someone else. In fact, he encouraged me to do that, independently as well as with the whole family. He said it might be good for me to do certain things for myself. But I didn't think it was a good time for me to be digging too deep into myself. There just wasn't enough of me to go around. Jeanette was the focus, and that focus is just now beginning to change a little.

That's why I asked the doctor if he would see me individual-

ly, from time to time, and
talk with him occasionally
him about Jeanette's ste
plays so many games, I j

There's a new wrinkle
me the other day that she
to ask the doctor about th
won't talk with him about
if she wants me to stop ju
all around, then I will co
about my feelings whe
considering going for family therapy

the parents and the
seemed so pointless
books out when
I think that
the release
Jazzerciz
Jazzer
and

that in the beginning of the stressful periods in our family,
Jeanette might not have become so terribly ill.

I know that I would have acted more quickly if I had had
more information before Jeanette became so sick. But once I
knew what was wrong, it was strange—I just couldn't read all
those books and listen to all those people on the radio and
television. I tried, but they all seemed to be blaming the
parents, or diet crazes. It was too much for me.

I did buy every book and article there was. But I didn't
finish reading any of them. Jeanette read every single one. In
fact, she diagnosed herself from those books. And Berton
read them all, after which he would quote from them extensively.
So I felt as if I had read them along with everyone else in the
house.

I just felt it wouldn't help to read all those different things.
Every case is so different, what would I learn? I might read
that someone developed anorexia because she had a family
that did her great harm. Then I would have to think about
that. And I didn't want to think about that. It was all I could do
to get through each day and hope that I could protect my
daughter from this special demon of hers.

I also wanted to avoid the guilt message in so many talk
shows and articles and books. Writers and talk show hosts
seem to like to assign blame, and their favorite targets are

families. I could not accept that. It
s, anyway. Actually, I think I threw all those
we moved a few months ago.

the one thing that really held me together was
and support I got in my exercise class. I go to
, and I love it. Throughout the whole nightmare,
ize was really important. That's the method of dance
exercise developed by Judi Sheppard Missett, and I give
er method a whole lot of credit. There were many days
when I felt physically and emotionally spent. So I would drag
myself to her class right here in Manhattan, and I could face
the rest of my problems. Just going through the classes
made me feel so much more positive and so much stronger.
The other members of the class always said the same sort of
thing I'm saying here. The class was everything from recreation to salvation.

Actually, I can honestly say that my family and my Jazzercize
classes were the only two sources of support I could find. Dr.
Sacker advised me that I could go to support groups, and
that the family might benefit from family therapy. But I
couldn't gather the energy to do any more than bring my
child back to the real world, and I still don't have the energy
for very much else.

From the beginning of the trips to Brookdale Hospital to the
doctor's office, there was nothing and no one in my life, or my
daughter's life, except the doctor, who understood and helped.
At first, I was deeply disappointed that the schools were not
more involved in identifying that Jeanette might be sick, or
need special help. Can you imagine being a school administrator or teacher, interviewing a student or working with that
student, and not checking with the child's mother when the
child looks so unhealthy?

Gradually, I have come to understand that schols are really
unprepared to deal with this. No one at any school she went
to ever checked to see what was wrong, or if her absences or
school problems were linked to any special need. As a matter

of fact, Jeanette has certain learning disabilities, which were never picked up in the whole time she was in elementary school.

The only reason why those learning problems were discovered was that she wanted to transfer from one school to another while she was in junior high, and she had to be tested. In New York City, a student can choose from a variety of schools, and she decided to attend a school that had a reputation for working successfully with children who required some extra help in order to earn good grades.

It was during that testing process that her disabilities were discovered. Even those records showed that she was consistently inclined toward certain learning problems from the beginning of her education. There are even records showing that I asked about those learning problems and was advised that she was performing well enough and would continue to improve over time.

No one ever discussed any special learning problems with me, I swear to you. I am the sort of parent who goes into action immediately to identify and correct any problem that I can see or understand. Learning needs can be handled within a very specific system. It's different from anorexia, which is so insidious and elusive in the beginning.

Anyway, I remember the meeting I had with the principal and the learning specialist. They told me she had a retrieval problem. Meanwhile, we were dealing with the weight-loss problems. I have to tell you, I had no idea what a retrieval problem was. But I had a friend who was a school psychologist, and I asked her what it meant later on that day. All she told me was that we all have retrieval problems sometimes, and she tried to laugh it off.

I was angry about the whole thing, and I didn't understand what the problem was, how it would effect her, or why it hadn't been identified and addressed earlier than seventh grade. All that came on top of the fact that Jeanette was clearly very sick at that time. When I was still very frightened, and still hoping that the weight situation would pass like any other teenage phase, there wasn't one teacher, principal, or counselor who called or wrote to ask whether Jeanette had any special needs at the time. That's when she weighed 80 pounds!

I would have welcomed a call like that. I know school people may have felt that I would go to them if I wanted help or input, but sometimes a parent just doesn't know what to say or how to begin. It's all so complicated. And I had lost confidence in them. They had failed to identify Jeanette's school-related needs. How could they help with a situation that didn't involve learning, which was supposed to be their specialty?

I can't say I'm angry at the school people, though. I had to sort of forgive them for failing to develop the right learning plan for her. And for avoiding the fact that Jeanette was acting more and more like she wasn't part of society at all. It was important to figure out where to go from that point, rather than to focus energy on trying to find out who was responsible for specific decisions made about my daughter. As I said, I had to forgive them. That way, I could direct all my thoughts toward helping my daughter....

When it comes to this topic, there's so much to say. I can't always tell what will or will not be valuable. It's hard to know what might be important to someone else. So I can only say what is important for me. It was important for me to hold my family together and save my daughter's life. The alternative was just unbearable. So I have had to keep on anticipating, balancing, and considering all the different needs that come up in my home—from my children, from my husband, and from inside myself. I feel right now that things are very positive. I said that before, but it's important.

Jeanette still has so many physical complaints. But she is improving. She still refuses to let us take a photograph of her unless she looks just perfect, by her standards. But it's easier to take because she's so much healthier all around. Of course, I wouldn't say that to her! You remember, she can't bear to hear that she looks healthy.

Actually, that's the final note to add. My success as a mother is that I don't talk out of turn. I'm resourceful. At this point, I have one main goal: to love my family well. Not perfectly, because I'm human, and perfection is impossible. But I can love them with all my heart, and learn to love them in a healthy way. I want to get to a safe, accessible place with my daughter, and I'm confident that we will succeed in that journey together. Because I'm getting better at problem-solving. And I'm good at waiting.

Jeanette can be confident that her mother will be there for her as she continues to heal. And her mother is ready to walk beside her as Jeanette tests out the world that she cut herself off from two important years ago.

Going back over the sequence of events was difficult for Sarah. So much had been compressed into two years that it felt more like five years as she started to recall first one incident, and then another. Even though dates and years were confusing at first, Sarah was very clear about the pattern her daughter followed in developing anorexia. First, there was always her intense effort to accomplish any goal she set. Then, Jeanette developed a new attitude toward her body; it would be perfect, no matter what she had to do to achieve perfection.

Sarah always understood perfection to be a relative condition for people. She never imagined that her daughter would relentlessly diet long after a reasonable goal weight had been achieved. But that is exactly what happened. Jeanette's passion for dieting developed quickly, as she focused all her energy on losing weight and looking different just at the time that she reached puberty.

Her pediatrician was pleased with that weight loss, because he thought it reflected a healthy self-control. That might have been a reasonable conclusion if the weight loss was considered in isolation. However, the weight loss had to be assessed more thoroughly. It was important to identify how long it took her to lose the weight, what type of diet she was using, whether she was exercising, and how much time or attention she was directing at those activities or issues.

Perhaps the most important point to establish would be whether she was content at an appropriate weight, or whether she was interested in continuing to diet, lose weight, and focus on food rituals. Closer questioning along these lines would have raised the pediatrician's concern, since Jeanette had lost 10 pounds over a period of just four weeks by living on a diet of no more than 800 calories a day. Jeanette was the only one who knew that at the time, though, and her pediatrician never asked.

At home, it seemed as though Jeanette were eating a healthy amount of food, primarily because she was sneaking much of her breakfast, lunch, and dinner to the family dog or into the folds of a napkin when no one was looking. Unless she had confided in a friend, no one would have been aware of her self-starvation in the very early stages. At least, not until she started to play bizarre food games. Those games involved listing foods she could eat and foods she couldn't, and the list was subject to constant change. She could sit for the full dinner hour just cutting and arranging food her mother had prepared. By the time everyone else had finished dinner, she would be just ready to begin.

The food games confused and even revolted her family, serving the purpose of diverting some initial attention from how little she was actually eating. By the time Jeanette's family understood that she was very sick, the bizarre behaviors had become part of her daily life, virtually the only topic of conversation between herself and her family. Sarah and Berton talked about the problem in the morning before Jeanette woke up, and in the evening, in hushed, tense voices, before they went to bed. The disorder was no longer a matter of weight and food. It was a family crisis that left each member of the family feeling isolated, misunderstood, resentful, and anxious.

So much of Sarah's experiences with doctors, schools, and family are familiar to all of us. You may already know how it feels to struggle to inform doctors unfamiliar with eating disorders, or some other problem regarding mental or physical well-being. You may already have experience struggling to work with school officials who might be unsure about how to approach you about sensitive and complex issues that could well be part of a growing-up phase for one of the hundreds of youngsters they see every day.

And you might have already begun to experience the rejections and confusing detours that can come up on the route to finding the right kind of help. But Sarah had two important things in her favor. First and most important, she recognized fairly early that her daughter's illness was not going to disappear, and that it was more than physical.

The second factor working in Sarah's favor was that she acted on that insight, and she refused to give up hope. That early recognition and affirmative attitude helped Sarah get Jeanette treatment before her eating disorder became more deeply entrenched. Jeanette had not yet lost more than a third of her normal weight. She had not developed a pattern of vomiting or laxative abuse, and she was not using any type of drugs to lose weight. Those facts helped speed her physical stabilization, since early intervention can make the critical difference in helping a person reach and maintain a healthy weight.

In part, it was Sarah's fast action that helped speed her daughter's physical stabilization. Now that Jeanette's health is no longer considered to be in imminent danger, her doctor can help her focus on getting in touch with her own feelings—a frightening but crucial stage for Jeanette. Sarah was able to help her daughter reach this increasingly healthy stage because she persisted in looking for the right help for her daughter. She understood that she and her daughter might have to interview doctor after doctor, therapist after therapist, before finding the right one for Jeanette.

Searching for the right kind of help can be time-consuming and difficult. When you get disappointed, angry, or just plain tired, it can be tempting to blame yourself, your child, teachers, doctors . . . everyone, if you do not find the help you need fast enough to offer relief at the moment you need it. The danger in that cycle is that you run the risk of getting so involved in blaming somebody that you might overlook the professional resources that can offer the help you expect and deserve.

Sarah's method was simply to forgive and move on. That may work for you, and it may not. Each person develops his or her own way to cope with the searching process. It was Sarah's way to get information, use it, and persist. She was uncertain about what anorexia actually involved, but one thing was clear to her: if she did not act quickly to secure help, she could lose her child forever. She was so afraid of losing Jeanette that it became possible for her to talk with strangers about this painful family secret.

Today, Jeanette, her family, and her doctor continue to work together to draw her gently back into the world outside herself. The future is unpredictable, but Jeanette's prognosis is good. At this point, Sarah, Berton, Margaret, and, most importantly, Jeanette, share that point of view. Now, the future means more to Jeanette than how much she can lose.

Anorexia nervosa is a persistent, insidious disorder that can develop slowly, over time. If you can recognize some of the symptoms that have been discussed so far, then you may be able to help the person involved get help before the illness progresses even further. So knowing the symptoms is an important part of being able to help. Knowing who might become anorexic or bulimic can also help. People who become anorexic or bulimic do not necessarily have a history of weight problems, and they do not have to be young or female. As you continue to read, you will discover that people can become locked into a cycle of food rituals that replace talking about feelings, or learning new ways to cope with stress and change.

6 | Rituals: Steven's Story

At 42, Steven Torman had a lifelong record of achieving every goal he set. He was accepted by the college he wanted most to attend. The woman he wanted to marry accepted his proposal, and he had two children who always worked hard to make him proud. He got the ideal teaching appointment in a top-ranking school district, and he lived with his family in the four-bedroom colonial that he had been determined to buy. He also weighed exactly 99 pounds.

There's one thing you have to understand right away. If I set a goal for myself, I make sure I achieve it. When I decide to accomplish something, the first thing I do is study it. I learn the rules of the game inside out. Then I play as if my life depends on winning. That doesn't mean that I'm everybody's image of a boy wonder. My God, I weighed 211 pounds when I was 18 years old. I was miserable at sports, and dating in high school was something the other kids did. But I wasn't trying to be an athlete or a lover in high school. I was trying to please my parents, and get the grades that would get me into the best school in the country.

My mother died when I was about 30, and my father retired to one of those planned communities in Arizona, but if you could talk with either one of them, they could tell you that I did please them, and I did get the grades. I made them proud when I got into Harvard, proud when Bonnie and I got married—I was always good at pleasing them.

I didn't have to go into therapy to know that I was afraid of disagreeing openly with anything they said or did or believed. I was always afraid of telling them if they upset me. As a matter of fact, I was never any good at letting anyone know what I really felt, good or bad. That wasn't just because I was afraid to make people angry at me. It was also because I never really knew how I felt. I would check to see how other people felt about things, and then I would decide that it was okay to feel like them and not okay to feel like me.

I can remember being about four years old, and watching how my sister would behave, and how my parents would react. My sister would be right in there, telling them out loud whenever she thought they were wrong, or whenever she was wrong. It was amazing. She acted as if she was totally confident that they would love her no matter what. And she still acts that way. She's incredible. We get along very well, by the way. We always have. But we really lived in entirely different worlds, emotionally. I have always tested out how everyone else felt about something before I could formulate an opinion of my own. Even about my own feelings.

This is a hard thing to understand if you haven't been there yourself. Think about spending your life guessing at what other people expect from you and then performing like crazy so they feel proud. Then, when they feel proud, it gives your life meaning. Without their approval, you really don't exist. It's a really stressful way to live, and all that stress can make you feel confused and angry. But you can't risk getting angry at anyone important to you, so you just keep pushing the feelings aside.

If it's hard for you to imagine life from that point of view, maybe it would help if you put yourself in my shoes. Imagine you're sitting at the dinner table with your parents and your older sister. You're a kid. Maybe you're five years old, or maybe you're 17. It doesn't really matter, because you haven't really grown up very much in your life. You may look older and get more done, but you still feel the same inside. You still feel powerless, unsure of yourself, and generally dependent on your parents or your teachers to tell you what is and is not good for you.

So there you are at dinner. As usual, there's more than enough food, because your mother and father agree that it's better to have too much than too little. That's understandable, since they both grew up in the Depression and remember going to bed hungry plenty of times. So there's more than enough for everyone to have seconds and even thirds. Plus dessert. You never have dinner without dessert, and you never get dessert without finishing every scrap of your dinner. Because it's a sin to be wasteful.

One of your parents always serves the dinner. That's an important food ritual in your house. You don't serve yourself, because the family rules are very clear: The children do not understand what kind of portions they should really have. So you pass your plate along, and it gets filled. You look forward to eating, because the eating helps distract you from any authentic feelings. You don't eat because you are hungry. You eat because it is time to eat, you've been told to eat, and eating makes you forget about any feelings that could be your own.

That means you eat to deal with how angry you are, because anger is one feeling that is definitely unacceptable in your family. Especially if you are a kid. So, you eat to deal with your problems. You eat all the food on your plate. You have seconds if you think you're expected to have seconds, and then you eat dessert. It doesn't matter whether you're full or not. In fact, you're not sure what it actually feels like to be hungry for a meal or a snack. You're just used to eating the amounts served at certain times, without exerting any control over what you eat, when you eat it, or how much you eat. And if your parents notice that you look preoccupied or if they think you have a problem, they thrust more food at you, and say the same thing every time: "*As long as you're eating, you're okay.*"

Inside yourself, you might be saying, "I'm not okay! I'm just eating!" But you never risk saying that out loud. Because food is so important to them. It's a symbol for being safe and powerful, and it helps remind them that they aren't poor anymore. You couldn't say that you felt differently even if you wanted too, because you don't really know how you feel.

You do know that too much food makes you fat. You also know that you have to buy your clothes in the husky department, and that your mother calls your potbelly and double chin cute. The kids in school have a different point of view. So you decide that those kids aren't supposed to matter. But you still feel bad. Can you imagine what life would be like in this environment? Your whole world at home and at school would revolve around the fact that you were fat.

My way of dealing with it in school was to laugh at myself before the other kids did, and to make sure that I was always the smartest kid in the class. That way, at least, the teacher had to pay attention to me. Even if he or she didn't like fat kids as much as the others.

Looking back now, I can see that the pressure of pleasing all of the grown-ups all of the time was incredible. I can understand now that it made me frustrated and angry. All I knew at the time was that I felt bad, and I couldn't tell anyone because I thought it was wrong to feel anything that my parents or teachers didn't feel first. I was also certain of one more thing: Food was an all-important weapon. If I wanted to make my parents anxious without actually getting angry, you can probably guess what I did. I would lose my appetite. That would upset them pretty badly. Especially my mother.

You see, if I didn't eat, it would make my parents nervous, worried, frustrated—everything I was feeling. And they couldn't actually get angry at me, because I wasn't doing anything wrong, so to speak. After all, if good little Steven had no appetite, how could he be punished? Having no appetite even for seconds or dessert was punishment enough in my house. It upset everyone and everything. I had actually figured out a way to get them upset without ever being direct about anything I was feeling.

I can see now that food was always a kind of weapon for me. I could use it to punish my parents, or to reward them. And I could use it to protect myself from finding out my own feelings. To this day, I still have a tendency to use food as a weapon. I have used it against my wife, even when I knew it was driving her out of her mind, and maybe even out of my life. I knew that my food rituals upset her, and I kind of enjoyed that. She would know it when I would vomit up a meal at home, and she would know exactly what my game was when I would pick for hours over a meal, never really taking a bite even if she had cooked for hours.

If someone you love is playing food games that make you feel angry, sick, or worried, then you know how difficult it is to cope with that person. You may get openly angry, and you may even insist that he or she stop or risk losing your love. Just as every bulimic and anorexic person is unique, so is every person who loves that person.

When you love someone who is bulimic or anorexic, you may find yourself in the same position as someone who loves an alcoholic: confused about what to do to help when the person you love seems to need you in ways that are complicated and often destructive. That's why it's important for you to get professional help and support in learning how to change the way you react to certain behaviors, so you can effectively help your loved one begin to understand and overcome the eating disorder. Steve's wife, Bonnie, found information, strength, and skills in the support group she attends for people whose lives are affected by eating disorders.

To this day she continues to struggle to learn how her husband's eating disorder is connected to the way he expresses anger, frustration, self-doubt, and confusion in regard to his own sense of self in his marriage, in his work, and in his private life, apart from family and other people or pressures. Bonnie believes that the appropriate treatment will help her husband learn how to truly manage his compulsion and overcome his need to purge, binge, and behave in a bizarre way to keep her at a distance.

At this point, she understands that Steve still finds intimacy threatening on a whole range of levels. He is anxious about sexual intimacy, and he finds it even more anxiety-producing to discuss his feelings, fears, and hopes with his wife. Slowly, he is getting used to the idea that she will accept him when he does discuss his feelings with her, no matter how confusing those feelings are. However, it's still difficult for him to believe that she will accept that anything he thinks or feels will be important or legitimate, just because it comes from him. So he tests her. He tests her to see if she really does love him, because he finds it so difficult to believe that *anyone* could love him.

It was always hard for Steve to accept that anyone could love him unless he was perfect. In his marriage, he has tested his wife's love extensively, by making himself almost impossible to reach and then looking to see if his wife was still making the effort to reach him. Steve and Bonnie are still married, and still living together, in part because they are working together to understand and defeat the eating disorder that nearly took Steve's life.

Bonnie says that she is grateful that her husband is still alive, and equally grateful that her support group is helping her learn how to help her husband continue to heal. Basically, Bonnie has come to terms with the fact that her husband continues to behave in ways that are designed to test the strength and integrity of their marriage. The progress that she has already seen gives her the hope and the strength to stay with him, to keep looking toward the future.

I know that my wife worried how it would affect the kids, and she was disgusted by purging. All I was interested in was upsetting her for upsetting me. Now, I never directly told her what she was doing that upset me. I wasn't really sure myself. I just knew I was frustrated and anxious, and I blamed her. I couldn't risk talking to her directly, mostly because I had no idea what to say. But I'm getting ahead of myself. I told you that I achieved every goal I ever set for myself, and I only got as far as my high school graduation. That was just the beginning.

You know, I got accepted into Harvard, and the family threw a huge party. Everyone was bursting with pride, but I have to tell you I wasn't. The only way I knew it was an accomplishment was because the rest of my family and all my teachers said it was. For me, it just meant that I had to set a new goal. I had to keep up that grade point average, and I had a new worry: girls.

If I was going to be a successful adult in the eyes of my parents, I would be expected to marry. I can remember, in the summer before I left for school, all the relatives were saying that I would meet one of those pretty girls who went to college to get married, and I would be married by graduation time because the girls would be able to tell that I would be successful. They kept saying that my brains would be my guarantee for success, and that meant I was a good catch. Well, I didn't believe that for a minute. I was fat. And girls who were looking for a good catch were not looking in the husky department, even at the exclusive Barney's men's store in New York, which is where my parents took me to buy my good suit for college.

The New Goal

Remember, in my life, reaching a goal just meant creating a new one. So you know that getting accepted to Harvard meant having to set a new goal. My family had already made it clear that I was supposed to get good grades, find the right girl, and go into teaching, because teaching was a job that was secure and respectable. Well, I already knew how to get good grades, and I was confident that I could figure out how to be a teacher. After all, I was good at school. The thing I had to work on was making myself attractive to the girls. So I immediately started to analyze the rules of that game. Especially since I had virtually no experience with girls.

Since there was no question that I would succeed in reaching my goal, the only question was how I would get there. From everything I could see, dating had to do with catching the attention of people who had no idea who you were. That meant that your appearance was everything, since it was the first thing anyone ever knew about you. So my first step was to plan to lose weight.

Losing weight at home would have been impossible without openly confronting my parents on just about every family routine and food ritual. But at school I could make my own rituals. I started to set specific, arbitrary rules about what I could eat, when I could eat, and how much I could eat. Just like my parents did. Only this time, I ate much less. I had never exercised in my life, so I didn't exercise to lose weight. I filled up my time studying, going to class, and dealing with food by either eating, planning to eat, or avoiding food entirely.

Basically, my strategy in the diet game was to eat very sparingly during the week and allow myself to eat and drink what I wanted on the weekends. I bought a scale, which I kept hidden under my bed. Not even my roommate knew that I had it. It was definitely not cool for a guy to have a scale in

his room, but I needed the positive reinforcement and structure it gave me.

Since I wasn't exercising, the one thing I knew I had to do
was count calories. I got a bunch of diet books, and in the
first two months of college, I lost 20 pounds. When I went
home for Thanksgiving, my parents almost dropped dead.
They thought I was starving. Actually, I had spent the week
before Thanksgiving fasting, because I knew I would have to
eat like a horse to please my parents. When I walked in the
door with my clothes hanging loose, my laundry in my
suitcase, and my A papers in a special file I made for my
parents, I knew all eyes would be on me. And I was prepared.

As soon as I walked in the door, I started to complain
loudly about how bad the cafeteria food was, and how much I
was looking forward to a good home-cooked meal. This way,
we could all blame the school for making me lose weight,
and I was off the hook! It worked like a charm. I was getting
this game down to a science. I was losing weight, and I was
still making everyone happy. That meant that I was safe. I was
also elated, because I was getting really good at a whole new
game: losing weight and keeping it off.

Anyway, in those four days at home, I must have eaten
more than I did anything else. They cooked me special
snacks, turkey surprises, and all kinds of gooey desserts
dripping with sugar and fruit. God, I can almost taste them
now. It was funny, though. I enjoyed sweets, but I can honestly
say that I never actually enjoyed food. I've realized recently
that I have never had a favorite dish. I just focused on eating.
Savoring a meal was never part of the process. I just focused
on eating.

During that first Thanksgiving weekend home from college, my family did two things together: eat and go Christmas shopping. I got my Christmas clothing gifts that weekend, because my parents were not going to let me go back
to school with clothes that did not fit. They told me in no
uncertain terms that they were not poor, and they would not

have me look like I couldn't afford to buy the proper clothes. Besides, how could I get the right girl if I looked like I couldn't afford to dress myself the right way? Notice, the message was not that I might be appealing or unappealing because of my weight, but only because of the fit and style of my clothes.

I went back to school looking better than I ever looked in my life, and I had managed to keep everyone happy at the same time. My goal was to reach 175 pounds by Christmas. That meant that I had another 14 pounds to go between Thanksgiving and Christmas, plus I had final exams and papers to finish. In order to reach that goal, I kept to the food rules I had set: Eat sparingly all week, let go on weekends, and then back to the rigid rules during the week. Like everything else I have ever set my mind to doing, it worked.

Part of the strategy was that my roommate would give me a reward. If I kept to my weight-loss schedule, he would set me up with a blind date—a girl who had never known me when I was really fat. I kept my end of the bargain, and he kept his. He set me up with a girl his date knew from school, and a whole bunch of us went out for pizza and a movie. That was the night I met Bonnie, except she wasn't my date. She was with some other guy, but we liked each other right away. Neither one of us wanted to be rude to the people we were with, but before the night was over, we had made plans to get together again alone.

I knew right away that I would really have to impress this girl, because she was terrific. Any guy would want to date her. She said she liked me because I was so smart, but I didn't believe her. I knew she wouldn't look at me twice if I was fat, but I never said anything like that out loud. That might make her dislike me, and then I'd be back to square one. And that was no way to play this game. You never went backwards. This girl was ideal, and I wanted to show her to my parents.

I hardly have to tell you, it was the best Christmas I ever gave my parents. I brought home a 4.0 average—straight A+—and a gorgeous girl who visited for a weekend and loved my parents right off the bat. They treated her like royalty, and all the time my father was winking at me like I had scored the hit of a lifetime. I knew I couldn't lose her then. Bonnie fit my family like a glove. She even ate enough to make my parents happy.

By the time the visit was over, I knew that she was the right girl for me. I can't tell you that I loved her, or that I love her now. I can only tell you that I knew she was the right one, because everyone else said so—even my roommate! So, with my weight at the target point of 175, my grades right where they were supposed to be, and my social life falling into place, I had to look for a new goal. I decided to get engaged at the end of my sophomore year, and the family put a lot of time, money, and effort into making a party in one of those halls that cost a fortune. You know—the kind with the giant crystal chandeliers and the different parties going simultaneously on all different levels.

The engagement party was bigger than some weddings I've been to, but all the parents pitched in, and they had a ball. Between school, part-time work, living far away from each other over vacations, and going on mostly group dates until we were engaged, Bonnie and I had every little time alone together. Sure, we had become intimate. We were planning to get married, and she was on the Pill. She was the first girl I was ever with, and she said I was her first guy. Who knows, of course.

Anyway, we were both so busy going through the basic steps of courtship, college, and part-time work, we never really took any time with each other. I don't remember even thinking about it. To tell you the truth, I don't know what we would have done if we did spend more time just developing our relationship. We probably wouldn't have gotten married. I can't say for sure. All I know is that we followed all the rules, graduated on schedule, got married that summer, and had our first daughter exactly twelve months later. Also on schedule.

I had been teaching fifth grade just one year when my first

daughter was born. Bonnie wanted to name her Sandra, and I wanted to make sure she also had my mother's name, so her full name is Sandra Ann. That way, Bonnie was happy, my mother was happy, and everyone was happy with me. I was learning fast. The rules for being married and supporting a family were the same as every other game. You figured out what was expected, and then you did it better than anyone else.

Everything went as expected. The kids are two years apart, first a girl and then a boy. They both look much more like Bonnie than like me, which they should be happy about. She really is terrific looking. I got tenure and then I got my master's, which meant that I was never really home very much. People think that teachers have nothing but time on their hands, but they're wrong. We're always going for extra courses, and we work all summer. I had a clamming business with a couple of other teachers, and the money we made was great. The hours were brutal, but it was okay by me. Lots of physical work, which helped me keep the fat off, and lots of time out of the house.

My own family was developing more or less like my whole life. Lots of milestones, lots of big gatherings and group activities, and plenty of messages that I was successful. When we bought a house, we didn't buy a starter house. I set the goal to buy a five-bedroom colonial, and I did it. That house is in a neighborhood with booming property values and a pool in every yard. I wanted to live and work in the same school district, so I could keep an eye on my kids' achievement. I succeeded in getting the house and the job I wanted, and Bonnie got involved right away in all that community service and PTA-type work. It was always good that way.

And if things were tight financially, I would just work more at clamming or tending bar, and I would cover the bills. I was determined that my wife, my kids, my home, my car— everything—would tell me that I had succeeded. When I pulled into my driveway at night, I would know that I was reaching those goals. If I didn't have all those things—wife, kids, house, new car every year—I wouldn't have been able to tell if I was successful. I really mean that. I needed markers, like you do when you're out on a boat. I needed those markers to tell me when I was safe, when I was at risk, and what I should do next.

So long as I could follow the markers and point to the milestones, nothing else mattered. So long as I had a new goal. Eating wasn't even a problem for me. I was true to my goal, never going under 174 or over 176 pounds. That was kind of a good game by itself, balancing out my weight so it stayed exactly where I wanted it. At my normal rate of activity, I could follow the same old ritual of eating lightly during the week, and eating and drinking anything I wanted during the weekends. It worked for me, so I had no fat problems. The kids were good in school, and Bonnie was busy with whatever she did, so I thought I should be okay. The problem was, it wasn't enough.

An extramarital affair was out. I never really liked sex to begin with, and the idea of having to deal with one more set of expectations was inconceivable, even though plenty of my friends were doing it. At that point, the country was just getting into its health kick. Natural foods were popular with lots of people, not just the hippies, whom I could never understand.

There was this one teacher in my school who was selling a whole line of vitamins, minerals—the works. It was wonderful stuff, and I know he never meant for me to disappear inside some sort of weird health fanaticism, but that's what I did. I decided that my new goal would be to change my eating habits to accommodate all this new information about health. My mother had died of a heart attack, and the doctor made it clear that the saturated fats and salty foods we lived by were the foods my mother died by. My father had to go on a new diet, too, so he was happy with all my new information. I had a whole new set of goals for myself and my family. At this point, I had not begun to vomit yet.

Eating Right to the End

Like every other goal I set, I immersed myself in learning how to eat the right way. I wouldn't eat sugar, and I reduced my intake of red meat. Processed cheeses were out, and the only bread in the house was seven-grain. I started a little garden in the back and got the family into eating the way I was. I bought vegetarian cookbooks and got my father on a diet regimen that he still says added years to his life and made him feel a thousand percent better.

I was really glad about that, but the truth was that *I* didn't feel any better. Fitness was a strange kind of goal. It seemed like you could never really reach it. It wasn't anything like getting the best grade possible, or buying just the right house. It was more elusive. And it was more disappointing. Everyone else was very impressed with my diet and health-food lifestyle, but I didn't think it was impressive.

Don't get me wrong. Plenty of other people told me I looked great, and that it was wonderful that I was helping my father. But for me, it was like the old Peggy Lee song, "Is That All There Is?" I was doing all these things that everyone said should make me feel better, but I didn't feel better. I would look in the mirror, and I wouldn't be satisfied. I was eating exceptionally well, but I didn't look exceptional. So I decided I had to lose weight.

I don't know quite why I decided that. But I do know that I would weigh myself at exactly the same time every morning and every night. The feeling I remember the most vividly was panic. I would panic before I set foot on that scale, because I was scared to death. Scared that all my effort to control my food intake would be for nothing. So I would build myself up to going on the scale, and then I would suffer an incredible letdown, because the outcome was never enough to make up for the effort.

As I see it now, it was a convenient game to play. If I spent a substantial part of my time at home building up to weighing myself, weighing myself, and then reacting to what the scale read, then I didn't have to deal with other things, such as being a father or a husband.

At that point, when I was getting totally involved in my weight-loss process, the opportunity came up for me to take a fully paid sabbatical, so that I could study something special. I jumped at the chance, thinking that a change would make me feel better. I didn't have to be enrolled in any special graduate school program in order to qualify. All the school district required was that I explore and report back to them on some new or developing aspect of elementary science education, which was a topic I particularly enjoyed.

Well, the sabbatical brought the biggest change in my life since I moved out of my parents' house. You see, being on sabbatical meant that I could make my own daily schedule. My life became totally unstructured, and I was overwhelmed at first. But I quickly decided that I would handle this change the way I handled every other challenge—by structuring every aspect of my day, and making myself comfortable again. So I started to run.

Basically, I would get up at 6:00 a.m., make coffee for myself, go out for a two-hour run, come home, shower, and then weigh myself. The whole process could take until about 11:00 a.m. because each step in the process was made up of very specific stages. Then I would leave the house and walk to various libraries or research centers. I would follow through on the sabbatical project, but I must say that I was devoting all my attention and interest to losing weight and building my ability to run longer and faster every day. And I had a new goal. I was determined to weigh 125 pounds.

I can't say that I deprived myself of any food every day of

the week. I would tank up on coffee, snack on vegetables and fruit, and be very careful to skip eating any real meals. Then, every Friday afternoon, just after I would finish my second run of the day, I would reward myself with the ugliest looking cakes you have ever seen. They would be dripping with sugar and fruit. Boy, that sugar was incredible. I was doing it just the way I planned, and I was not vomiting. Yet.

Well, if you know anything about basic health, you know that if you run your brains out, skip main meals, drink coffee like it was water, and gorge yourself on cakes that are almost 100 percent sugar, you're going to hurt your body. In my case, I got a cardiac arrythmia. That's when your heart beats at peculiar rates, and the doctor puts you in the hospital. That scared me. My mother died from heart disease, and here I was, in the same hospital where she died.

As I'm talking to you now, it's hard for me to believe that I was so relentlessly self-destructive. But when they signed me out of that hospital, I took the arrythmia and the scare tactics from the doctor, and I turned them into a challenge. I had set a goal for myself: 125 pounds. And I was going to reach it. But I knew that the dieting and the running alone wouldn't get me there. I had to understand more about nutrition, chemical balances necessary for the heart—everything to play both sides of the fence. Because that's what I did. I studied the literature on cardiovascular training, strength training, and nutrition, and I did it all to the most extreme limits possible. There was no way that I would be happy until I reached 125 pounds. Then I would stop.

Sometimes, I felt I might die. Not from losing weight, but from failing to lose weight. So I joined a health club in order to use the sauna, and I played the same game as the dancers and the jockeys. I would sweat off water weight, jumping from the sauna to the cold shower, on and off, for a total of one hour in the steam. That helped get down the weight, so my weigh-in sessions were getting increasingly intense, exhilarating, and important.

But one victory meant another defeat. I was losing strength, so the running was getting more difficult. But it didn't matter. Nothing and no one else mattered. Only the rituals. The running, dieting, sauna sessions, weigh-in episodes, were all elaborate and intricate rituals. And I was perpetually seeking new ways to increase strength and still lose weight—different strategies that I could incorporate into my regimen. I would read, talk with people, listen to radio talk shows, and watch television programs, all to gather new information and ideas so I could reach my goal, and be happy.

You see, in my mind, I had never really experienced any kind of success that I could actually feel on my own. I always needed someone else to help interpret my experiences, so I would know what to feel. I could count on my family and the people at work to do that for me, to a point. Now my friends and family have stopped all that interpreting—they expect me to interpret my feelings, and other messages from other people, on my own. But at that point, I was completely into the weight-loss game, just like the dancers and the jockeys. Sweating off water weight by jumping from the sauna to the cold shower helped get down the weight on the scale. Of course, it doesn't do a single thing to help you lose fat, but at that point, I didn't care. I was losing weight a little more rapidly, adding zest and importance to my appointments with the scale.

What's important here is that I always needed someone else to interpret my experiences, so I would know what to feel. I could count on my family, my colleagues, and my students for some of that. But I wanted more. I wanted people to look at me and see something special. I wanted to look in the face of a stranger and see admiration, so I would know that I accomplished something that was just about impossible for most people, especially in our society.

Think about it. What's the one thing that everyone's got too much of and no one can lose? Weight. That's right. Everyone's always trying to lose weight. But very few people really succeed in reaching their goal. From what I've seen, more people fail at losing weight than at any other single goal. I found out how to do what everyone else couldn't. I could lose as much or as little weight as I wanted. And that meant I was better than everyone else.

Up until that time, I had not yet vomited. And I had not yet reached my goal of 125 pounds. Then I saw a television talk show about bulimia. I didn't watch it and say, "Wow! That is disgusting and dangerous behavior that I should stay away from." I watched and said to myself, "Boy, that sounds interesting. I can see that I'll actually be able to eat again."

So that's when it started. I ate my first full meal in months, went up to the bathroom, and threw it all right back up. It wasn't long before I couldn't take the feeling of satiety at all, and that feeling could come from the least amount of food or drink. You know how every dieter in the world drinks Perrier? Well, that's partly because it's pure and partly because the natural carbonation helps you feel more full, more satisfied. Well, I quickly reached the point where drinking just a small glass of Perrier would make me feel that I had gained ten pounds. I couldn't concentrate on anything or anyone. I just had to get rid of the feeling as soon as it came over me.

So I would vomit. And immediately after vomiting, I would feel relief. Deep, abiding satisfaction and relief. Best of all, I would feel powerful. I didn't have to look to anyone else to see if I had accomplished something special. I knew. I was doing this thing that other people just couldn't handle. I was eating the way I was expected to, but I wasn't gaining weight, because I was able to do the most difficult thing of all—vomit the dinner that all the other people had to hang on to psychologically, physically, because they just didn't have the strength to do what I did. Every day, and every night. And I didn't throw up into the toilet. I thought that was demeaning. I threw up in the shower, so that I could clean myself inside and out. Totally.

I was genuinely proud of this thing I was doing. Sure,

people were lecturing me, but their opinions didn't really matter. I decided they were jealous, and I wouldn't let them near me. I was on a total high, and I felt that I had finally achieved absolute power. Since I was a very well educated student of nutrition at this point, I learned everything I could about potassium levels, electrolytes, cardiovascular function, metabolic rate—everything I thought I needed to know about how to keep your system in a state of technical biochemical balance.

Looking back, I know that I was just avoiding the truth. Denying the reality that I was gravely ill, and that I was risking my life every time I decided to vomit. I would look in the mirror and I would say to myself, "Okay, self. You're thin. So what. That's what everyone in America wants to be. Enjoy it!"

I was out of touch with the fact that I was compelled to vomit. Out of touch with the fact that I was just living to get high, like a common junky. Me. Everyone's perfect Steven. The day this perfect Steven weighed in at 125, I can tell you this: I felt like I had finished a marathon, won the lottery, and got elected to the Presidency of the United States, all in the same day. I was totally euphoric, and I felt more powerful than I had ever felt before. That was the beginning of what was very nearly the end of my life.

When Power Turns to Panic

Once I reached 125 pounds, I knew I could do anything. It didn't satisfy me. It was the encouragement I needed to push on. In the year that I had been on sabbatical, I had achieved what no one at my school could believe. Oh, I gave the administration my research report, which they received very well. But no one could stop talking about how thin I was. They were absolutely amazed by what I had been able to accomplish. The women were absolutely dying for my secret. It was great, at first.

Maybe all the attention made me feel impervious to failure. I'm not sure. But all of a sudden, I was bingeing. Three thousand, even five thousand, calories inside of a half hour, parked in my car in the teachers' lot. Then locking myself in the private, single-stall men's room, vomiting for the other half of my lunch hour, and walking back into class feeling completely in control. You know how you feel when you finally accomplish something that you thought you might never achieve? Well, that's how I felt when I mastered bulimia.

I was actually able to do anything, and eat anything, and still lose weight. I didn't even have to run as much! So I thought, Why not binge? Other people did it and they looked fine to me. I wouldn't have to skip any meals, or let anyone else know what I was doing. I genuinely felt that anyone who got sick doing this was just bad at it.

So there I was, feeling superhuman, eating gallons of ice cream, pastries, nuts, anything that I used to forbid myself to eat on weekdays. I would revel in the fact that I could eat exactly what I wanted, when I wanted, and never gain an ounce. As long as I was still losing weight, I didn't care about anything else. And I kept losing weight, because I kept on working it off and working it out. My body didn't show the results of a single calorie, and I was proud of that. My food rituals were getting increasingly elaborate and secret, and I took comfort in the structure and focus they gave my whole life.

There were just a few problems that were beginning to get to me, through all my defenses and rituals. First of all, a lot of people were beginning to stare at me. The kids at school, my colleagues, people in shopping malls . . . everywhere I went, people stared. And they whispered to each other as I passed. That made me a little bit self-conscious. So I thought, well, maybe my family and friends are right. Maybe I've gone a little too far. There was just one problem. I couldn't stop.

* * *

As Steve continued to be consumed by his disorder, his family began to develop different ways of coping with the fact that something was terribly wrong. No one in the family realized that bulimia was a disorder that could be treated. As Steve became progressively more involved with food and exercise compulsions, his family worked industriously to try to keep the family as normal-feeling as possible. They were intensely concerned that no one find out this awful secret. They individually and collectively lied to cover up the fact that Steve might spend hours at a time purging, or six hours just doing different aerobic exercises.

Each family member coped in a different way. Mostly, they felt that if they continued to behave as if nothing was wrong, Steve would get through what they saw as an overinvolvement in health and fitness, and would get back to being the Steve they understood and could predict. Sometimes, family members would get angry at Steve, and explosive arguments would erupt, particularly when the family were gathered together for some special occasion or holiday. But the arguments were so intense and painful, they only served to demonstrate to the family that it did not pay to even discuss their feelings, since every honest discussion was doomed to go out of control.

Now, as the family continues to receive support-group guidance, and Steve remains in therapy, it has become clear to each of them that Steve will continue to change, and that he will never be the man they used to find so predictable and controlled. However, they are all relieved that treatment has helped Steve begin to change his behavior for the better, and they are hopeful that the changes will continue.

While Steve has learned how to change, the family has undergone a similar process. No one covers things up for Steve, and no one protects him from his work or the people he loves. The entire family has learned to become interdependent in the way each member loves and empowers the others, and Steve is held accountable for his actions for the first time. It is not the same as pressuring him to be perfect. It is simply expecting him to express his feelings and needs in a way that makes it possible for other family members to respond accordingly.

When Steve finally understood that he was out of control, he was able to accept medical and psychological help more readily than if he were still in denial about how bulimia was controlling him. Accepting the fact that his body was controlling his behavior was a terrible moment of realization for Steve. It was at that moment that his sister saw his panic and gave him the information he needed to find help, so he could help himself.

When I found out I really couldn't stop, I was paralyzed by fear. I hope that you can appreciate how overwhelming that truth was. It finally occurred to me that I was totally out of control. There was no way I could stop vomiting. If I so much as drank a glass of water, I would panic at the feeling of the fluid in my stomach. I had to expel it. And I would push anyone and anything aside in order to accomplish that goal. I'm not sure if the panic was a consequence of my fear of gaining weight, or if it was an emotional issue of power and control. I'm still working that out in therapy. But I do know that I was down to just two feelings: panic and power. That is when I realized I was in serious trouble.

You may think I should have figured that out much earlier. After all, I was a grown man, and I weighed exactly 99 pounds. I should have been able to look in the mirror and see that I was desperately ill. But when I looked in the mirror, all I really saw was a man who had been able to master all the rules of the game of weight loss and food management. I was really proud of what I had done to myself. I enjoyed how much it upset my family, and I felt that the people who said they were the most concerned were just jealous.

There were just two things that I had not counted on. First of all, I could not stop vomiting. That was devastating, because a major motivating thrust behind the choice to vomit was that it made me feel so powerful. When your weapon turns on you and takes on a power of its own, it's time to get rid of it. Only I couldn't. And that was scary.

I'll tell you the other thing I hadn't counted on. I stopped losing weight, and I started to gain. You may think, well, that's a good thing. Think again. Right now, while you're reading, think of something that really makes you panic. Maybe it's being alone at night on the subway. Or it may be heights. You could be afraid of being locked in small, dark places. Or you may fear losing a child or someone else you love. You get the idea. There has to be at least one circumstance or condition in life that would leave you in a state of panic, and if you imagine yourself in that condition, then you will understand how I felt when I realized I could no longer lose weight at will. I panicked.

During my whole involvement with weight loss, food abuse, and bulimia, I had never been to a doctor. I figured that I knew what they knew, because I read the same books. In fact, I really felt that I knew more, because I was able to do what they said could not be done safely. Well, my sense of omnipotence was quickly giving way to total panic, and my sister picked up on the fact that I was changing.

Now she says that she had been watching me carefully, waiting for the moment when it seemed that I had run out of weapons, even temporarily. She sensed my panic, and she gave me the name of Dr. Sacker. It seems that she saw him on television, and she experienced this huge sense of relief. There was a doctor on TV who was talking about this thing that her brother had! Better yet, he was saying that it wasn't just something that afflicted ballerinas and other young women. She wrote his name and number in her personal phone book, and then she started her subtle campaign of waiting for me to have a vulnerable moment. I can say now that I'm more than grateful to her. I owe her my life. I only wish she had been able to see just one of the thousands of vulnerable moments I had before that time when she sat me down in her living room and gave me Dr. Sacker's name and number.

Anyway, I think she handled the whole thing really well. She told me later that she had called Dr. Sacker at his office before she gave me his number, and had told him that she thought I was dying. When she told him that I had a history of weight problems and that I was looking more skeletal every day, he told her that I was suffering from a disease that could kill me if it wasn't stopped. That was all she needed to hear. She saw how frantic and haunted I was looking, and she decided it was now or never. Well, I have to tell you, I didn't jump to the telephone and call Dr. Sacker for help. Going for help to anyone was very difficult for me. For me, it was always a very clear sign that I had failed at doing something on my own.

I took the piece of paper with the doctor's name and phone number, and I folded it, carefully and repeatedly, until it was very small. Then I tucked it into a tight section of my wallet, next to my emergency money, and I waited. I waited two weeks. When the panic became overwhelming, and I could no longer control my weight or my need to vomit, I gave in to reality, and I called Dr. Sacker.

I was really disappointed that he wasn't available to talk with me right away when I called the first time. I was hurt and annoyed, and I hung up. But I called back later the same day, and I made an appointment. You know how alcoholics can experience a sense of hitting bottom? It's the feeling you get when you know that you can go no lower, unless you go to your grave. That's the feeling that I had. So I made the appointment, and I showed up 15 minutes early.

A New Feeling of Power

In some ways, you can compare bulimia to alcoholism. It's a progressive disease, and it will kill you if you don't stop your own self-destructive behavior. The only difference is that the alcoholic has one concrete opportunity not available to the bulimic. The alcoholic must abstain from drinking any alcohol. Period. No one can abstain from eating. So the bulimic has to eat, yet abstain from behavior that revolves around eating. It's incredibly difficult. You have to start learning how to eat all over again, as if you were a very small child. From my point of view, you have to be highly motivated to change.

I'll tell you what motivated me. I walked into Dr. Sacker's office, introduced myself, sat down, and waited. He looked me straight in the eye and said, very simply, "If you want to die, there's the door. I can't help you. If you want to live, we can work together."

That was great. This was the first time someone who could have taken over all the power in a situation actually shared power with me and let me know that I had a major responsibility for making the process work. He didn't say, "Don't worry. I can take care of you." His message was that I could take care of myself, and he could help me acquire the skills and attitudes I would need to help myself.

Like a sober alcoholic, I count the months that I have been able to eat, drink, work, deal with my family, and sleep without bingeing or purging. It's been 13 months and 10 days. But for the first six months of treatment, I continued to vomit. And I would come into the office and tell him that I was still vomiting. I was waiting for him to fail my test for people in charge. I was waiting for him to take over, get disappointed, or show that he was revolted by me. But he didn't do any of that. He didn't get upset with me. He was just concerned. Then I realized with a shock that he wasn't playing my game. I could not upset this person by vomiting, abusing laxatives, or eating 5,000 calories in a single sitting.

He would say things like, "Well, try not to vomit as much," or, "What were you feeling just before you decided to binge?" I was playing the rebellious teenager, and he was refusing to play the anxious and aggravated parent. That left me without a real role to play, and it was becoming increasingly clear that, in Dr. Sacker's office, there was no game to play.

Healing was an important process that was not a game, and the sooner I took responsibility for what happened to me, the sooner I would feel better. That message came through loud and clear, and it made me feel excited, affirmative, and scared to death.

He had mentioned the drug Parnate to me, as a form of treatment that has helped some people stop purging. But he said that I wasn't ready for it yet. He would not just prescribe a drug. I had to accept responsibility for my actions and know that the drug would just help me with my impulses. I would still be in charge of my behavior. Well, I understood that to mean that he felt I wasn't in charge of my actions, and that really annoyed me. After all, I'm not dumb. I knew I really could die. I could suffer a stroke or cardiac arrest. I could get irreversible problems with my digestive system, my colon... my whole body could start shutting down. So I set a goal. I decided that I would prove to Dr. Sacker that I was ready for Parnate.

You already know how I am with goals. I succeeded in proving myself, and I got the prescription. That day I went home, took the prescribed amount, and that was the first day in years that I did not vomit. And I haven't vomited since.

Of course, I read as much as I could about the drug. It's only given to profoundly depressed people, which made me feel good, in a perverse kind of way. It showed me that I was really sick, and that I could be treated. I'm not on that medication anymore, by the way. But it gave me the chance to gather my physical strength, break the cycle of bingeing and purging, and start to deal with the emotional issues that made me so self-destructive and out of touch with my feelings.

It's been a long road for me, and I have a long way to go. I'm a perfectionist, and when you're a perfectionist, you have to suffer from low self-esteem. There's no way you can ever live up to your own expectations, because you can never be perfect. So you punish and destroy yourself, but you're not quite ready to just jump off a bridge. So you pick a slow process of destruction, and withdraw into it, perfecting your ability to cause yourself harm.

With Dr. Sacker, I've been able to go through a different process: slowly becoming healthy. I can't say I'm getting back to health, because I don't think I was ever there. I had no frame of reference for feeling good about myself, and I had no idea how to play the game of wellness. I've been learning, slowly, that wellness is not a game at all. It's a way of life, and it's the only choice.

Don't let me kid you. The road to recovery has not been smooth. As soon as I stopped vomiting, I stopped all the compulsive exercise. That meant that I immediately gained weight. Think back again to whatever it is that scares you, and then magnify it a thousand times. I was terrified, at first. And I sabotaged treatment right and left. But my fear of dying overcame my fear of gaining and my need to vomit. I can honestly say that gaining weight annoys me now, but I don't panic. I've overcome the fear, anxiety, and self-hatred, and I simply problem solve. It's a whole new feeling of power, and it makes me feel better about everything.

Today, I still have difficulty sitting down and eating a whole meal. But I do attempt it. I'm getting reacquainted with my family, and they have been phenomenal. My kids and wife have also been to see a counselor, to help them understand that the things I did had nothing to do with them, and everything to do with me. I feel as if I had spent my life on an extensive journey into a region where communication was virtually impossible. Now I'm back from the journey. I'm on entirely new ground, and I like what I see, even when I look in the mirror.

Steven Torman's story illustrates one of the most important aspects of eating disorders like anorexia and bulimia. Each individual person who suffers from anorexia, bulimia, or bulimarexia is unique. Age, sex, symptoms, eating behaviors, and physical activities can vary. There are only two factors that appear in every story: a desperate need for control and an equally desperate impulse toward self-destruction.

Because each individual bulimic or anorexic person is unique, it's important to understand that symptoms, activities, and eating habits can vary widely. If you want to know more about signs that indicate that you or someone you care about may be suffering from anorexia or bulimia, the next chapter is for you. You will be able to hear from people suffering from anorexia or bulimia. And you will be able to hear from the family members, friends, and doctors who observed the problems, and tried to help.

III

THE PROCESS OF HEALING: TREATMENT THAT WORKS

7 | What Treatment Involves: Understanding the Process

Treatment is a very hard concept to consider if you don't feel sick. It took me four months of dealing with some very serious physical problems to admit that the physical problems were connected to my bingeing and purging. If I was going to live, I had to start changing. And I needed to find someone who knew it would take me time to give this thing up, because it was all I had. I needed to get something else in exchange. I just couldn't stop without filling the void that would be left in my life. But I wanted my life. Looking back, I can see how I had to get over my fear, understand how I got sick, and then allow someone to help me figure out how I could help myself....I know I'm alive today because my doctor stood by me, and I trusted him.

—Paula Crowell, age 26
Recovering bulimic

Treatment for any problem is simply professional guidance that helps you accomplish the very difficult task of changing. From the day you first think about looking at the different options you have to receive professional guidance and support, you are going through the process of finding help. You have already seen how problems of powerlessness and poor self-image can precipitate problems with eating disorders for children and adults. When issues of personal power and self-image are involved, treatment must empower those individuals to test their strength and to consider alternative self-concepts.

This entire section covers key aspects of treatment philosophy, process, and practice, when treatment involves building a positive self-image based on information, strength, and confidence.

Getting Over the Fear

Ordinarily, finding help is not as simple as seeing the problem, picking up the phone book, finding a number, calling for help, and finding it right away. Most often, finding the right guidance or information takes time, and you may have to just think about it for a while. The idea of changing can make you feel extremely anxious, even if you are thinking of changing for the better. With that understanding, you can readily see that it may be very difficult and stressful for bulimic, anorexic, or bulimarexic people to seek help without carefully thinking about it first.

Imagine how you would feel if your mother, father, sister, brother, spouse, or even your doctor told you today that you must see a special doctor to deal with your weight and eating problems. If you are bulimic or anorexic, you probably feel that what you eat, when you eat, and how you eat it is the one thing in life you can count on controlling. Now someone is telling you that you must go to a doctor who will try to make you give up the one thing in your life you think is guaranteed to make you feel confident and strong.

The first thing you may want to do is escape. The only problem is that escape requires some sort of confrontation or open refusal to do something that does not actually involve food. That kind of confrontation may be virtually impossible for you if you are convinced that the one power you can wield is the power of eating or not eating, depending on how you feel.

Since running away may seem impractical or impossible, you may choose a different kind of escape: finding out what the doctor expects, doing it precisely, and giving the appearance of healing in order to get rid of the doctor as soon as possible.

If you have medical or social problems because of your eating disorder, you may decide to go to a doctor on your own, and that may impress the doctor and the other people who care about you. If you agree to go for help, the other people in your life may interpret your apparent willingness as a sign that you are clearly and genuinely concerned with healing. You may share their interest in overcoming the disorder. On the other hand, your decision to go for help may be a sign that you want the doctor to help you get rid of any uncomfortable, embarrassing, or painful problems caused by starving, bingeing, or purging.

You may go to a doctor for any number of reasons. Someone may make you go, or you may go to please someone else. You may want a doctor to help you get rid of some symptoms of your eating disorder, or you may be hospitalized with physical problems that have developed as a result of your eating disorder. It's also possible that you have reached the point where you want to get the help you deserve in understanding and defeating your eating disorder.

One or more of those reasons may motivate you to go to the doctor's office and to remain in treatment until you achieve your goal. Charlotte Wesley recalls what she felt when she finally agreed to go to the doctor after having been anorexic for nearly eight months:

I went partly because I wanted to get my family off my back, and partly because I wanted to see what the doctor could tell me that I did not already know. I actually wondered if he could tell me new tricks or ideas about how to lose weight or eat differently. I remember feeling incredibly anxious when they made the appointment. In fact, I kept making different plans so that the appointment got put off for three weeks, until the pressure from my family got impossible, and I made time to really go to that doctor.

Once I admitted to myself that I had to go, I concentrated a lot of energy on figuring out how to prove that no stupid doctor could make me change, any more than my family could make me change. I decided that I was in charge, and no one was going to push me around and manipulate me. I would manipulate them first. It's hard for me to believe it now, but I know I rehearsed what I would say, what the doctor might say, what I would say back—it helped, doing all that, because I was scared to death. When I concentrated on planning what to do and how to do it, I could put the fear in perspective, because I was doing something constructive to protect myself from the person I was most afraid of: the doctor.

My mother was the one who drove me to the doctor's office. I know she was talking the whole way there, but I can't remember a thing she said. All I can remember is that I was actually shaking with fear. The anxiety was unreal. All I could think about was how I could make this situation work to my advantage. How could I get by, satisfy the family for a while, and get this doctor to leave me alone.

To control my nerves, I concentrated on developing a strategy to pacify the doctor. I figured the only way any doctor would really leave me alone would be if I listened to every single word he said. That was the bottom line. I decided to give him the impression that I was the most cooperative thing on two feet, so he'd be happy. I knew he would love that. You see, I'm an expert at making people happy. It doesn't take me long to figure out how to play by someone else's rules. In this case, I was playing for control over my life. That's how I felt. You can't have bigger stakes than that. So I had to win.

After our first meeting, I figured I had him in the palm of my hand. He said I had to agree not to lose another ounce, so I agreed. I would have agreed to anything. My mother had already told him I was going to the spa every day, plus running five miles a day, and he told me that I had to stop running until I stabilized at a weight that he called "healthy for me." He also said that I should temporarily suspend my trips to the spa, too. I remember seething inside as he told me that, but I agreed. I figured, okay, I'll find some other way to work off calories, but I never said that out loud. If I did that, I might alienate him, and if I did that, I was afraid he might stick me in a hospital.

Actually, I felt like I was in a war, and I was taken prisoner by the enemy. So I thought about scenes like that in the movies, where the prisoner just gives name, rank, and serial number. Then, if the enemy keeps on pushing, the prisoner may have to give them a little more, to make them happy. Act like you give in, but keep the fight going on the inside. And that's exactly what I did. I kept that fight going on the inside, where I always did most of my fighting, anyway. So I was good at it.

Feeling anxious about going to a medical doctor or psychologist is perfectly normal. The anxiety or fear may cause a whole range of symptoms, such as muscle tension, elevated blood pressure, difficulty concentrating on tasks, headache, stomachache, or a variety of other physical or emotional reactions that typically come up when you feel anxious or fearful.

No matter whether you go to the doctor for a checkup, or for help with a specific problem, you may feel nervous about going, and you may procrastinate for a while before actually going. If you have a secret that you want to keep from the doctor, or if you are afraid that the doctor will take away your freedom or something else you consider precious, you will probably feel more than anxious or fearful: You may feel extremely defensive.

Feeling defensive is also normal when you have a secret you want to keep hidden. Whether you binge, purge, starve yourself, or engage in a combination of extreme eating habits, you may feel compelled to do anything to hang on to the freedom to practice those eating behaviors. Just the way smokers or drinkers may hide their behavior from family or friends who assert that abusing alcohol or cigarettes is self-destructive, bulimics and anorexics often hide their food rituals from people who would try to make them stop. If you are bulimic or anorexic, and you are on your way to see a doctor, you become as defensive as Charlotte Wesley, because your first interest may be in getting that doctor out of your life, so you can continue to engage in the behavior that the doctor is likely to diagnose as self-destructive.

All that anxiety, fear, and defensiveness is normal in the beginning of your relationship with the doctor. After all, you want to hang on to the behavior, and the doctor wants you to stop. It's hard to believe that you can stop the starvation, the bingeing, or the purging. It's hard to imagine that anything else could make you feel so safe and so secure.

Charlotte certainly experienced all those feelings of anxiety, fear, and defensiveness. She was desperately afraid of becoming fat, and she was determined to fight her doctor virtually to her own death, so long as she could keep her grasp on the one thing she could call her own: her unswerving ability to deny herself the food that other people could not resist, and the resulting joy she felt when people stopped, stared, and commented on how thin she looked.

Since that first meeting, Charlotte has made enormous strides toward healing. Her weight has stabilized at an acceptably healthy level, and she is willing to spend her sessions discussing feelings rather than focusing on food, eating habits, or exercise strategies. In fact, she is increasingly able to make appropriate, constructive decisions about complex and confusing situations in life, such as choosing a college or going out on a date. The more skilled she becomes at making choices and decisions in complex situations, the less likely she will be to retreat into extreme food and exercise games that used to give her a sense of control in a confusing and complicated world.

Like I said, I was scared to death, in the beginning. I defended myself all kinds of ways. Mostly, I would just do exactly what I was told, or act as if I was doing exactly what I was told. Over a few months, I started to trust the doctor a little bit more every session. I think I started to trust him because he didn't try to fight with me. He just suggested different ideas to consider and left me with the choices. It's hard to express, but basically I know I was always in control. He wasn't interested in taking control over what I did or when I did it. He just wanted me to commit to following some basic steps that he said would keep me out of the hospital. And he was right. I followed those steps to the letter, and I was never hospitalized. Now, I can actually let go of some of the eating rituals and the starvation, because I'm taking control over some of the things that used to scare me as much as anything could scare me in the world.

Charlotte's initial fear, anxiety, and defensiveness have given way to a sense of confidence and positive self-control that continues to develop every day. There are days when she slips, gets anxious, grasps for the familiar comfort she derived from denying herself food, but the slips are fewer and farther between all the time. Basically, Charlotte responded to a treatment approach built on the understanding that anorexic and bulimic people often require a highly personalized combination of support, challenge, and security before they are willing to risk looking for comfort and gratification any other way. Each individual suffering from anorexia, bulimia, or bulimarexia is different, requiring different degrees of safety and structure before he or she even attempts to give up the food games. Before agreeing to allow her story to be told here, Charlotte insisted that she be able to share with you how she felt on the day she calls her turning point:

I know that every week I would say things, and the doctor would say things, and I would try to keep one step ahead of him—always trying to outsmart him. And if he said or did something that made me furious, I would get even. Like the time he went away on vacation for ten days, just after I reached my goal weight to go back to the health club. I finally figured out that I needed him, and he left. One side of me knew that he didn't leave forever—just for ten days. But the other side was enraged. The voice inside me that helped me keep the rest of the world at bay won out, and I decided I would lose ten pounds—one for every day he was gone—just to remind him who was really in control here. I lost ten pounds, right to the ounce. When he came back and saw I had lost weight, he was very matter-of-fact about the whole thing. I remember thinking, "There, you bastard. I win! I win! Show how upset you are!" But he didn't look upset at all. He just asked me how I felt about losing the weight. I remember looking straight at him, wanting to say I felt great, but just feeling pain. And loss. Intense, profound loss. Here was the first person I couldn't control by eating or starving, and I remember feeling utterly empty—like I wanted to die. That's when it happened. I actually could feel the turning point. He knew that I was going through a loss and grieving as intense as what you go through when someone you love dies suddenly. That's when he zeroed in with the best support anyone can offer: the understanding that if you yourself are strong enough to deny yourself food even when you are constantly, horribly hungry, then you are strong enough to do anything—even throw the hunger away.

At that point, I started to consider the possibilities out there. My God! I could do anything I wanted. I didn't have to wait to see if someone else was happy or sad about what I did. I could just check with myself. For the first time in my life, I could really just check to see what I felt about something. Ever since that day, I check with myself all the time.

And I have to tell you, I love it. Sometimes it's scary, but at least I know I'm in charge. I don't have to look at anyone else to see what I'm supposed to feel. And I know that strength to reach a goal or understand my feelings comes from me. Not the doctor. Not my father. Not my mother or my boyfriend. Me. Sure, they can give me input. But I'm the one who has to handle the choices, so I'm the one with the control over what I feel or do. And that control beats all hell out of pain and starving.

8 | Personal Power: One Key to Treatment That Works

If you were to attend a meeting where some people were bulimic, some were anorexic, and some were both, you would discover that each person is unique in the way he or she has developed, maintained, or fought the disorders. Just as there are no two people with identical fingerprints, there are no two bulimic, anorexic, or bulimarexic people who are the same.

On the other hand, a fingerprint has certain essential characteristics that make it possible for you to identify it in a general way. Once you can identify a fingerprint, then you can do what you choose: You can wipe it away, make a copy, research it, connect it to someone—anything you want. The same basic concept applies to eating disorders. Even though people with anorexia, bulimia, or bulimarexia are different from each other, they also share certain basic characteristics. It is those shared, fundamental characteristics that make it possible to develop treatment approaches that have been very successful in helping people understand and defeat anorexia, bulimia, and bulimarexia.

When Every Night Is Opening Night: The Pressure of the Perfect Performance

No matter how many other special, individual issues preoccupy each bulimic, anorexic, or bulimarexic person, all people with these disorders tend to share a common struggle for personal identity. It is true that we all get confused about who we are and why we do what we do, especially when we go through periods of change. All through infancy and childhood, we normally experience opportunities, successes, and frustrations that help us grow and discover ourselves, and the world outside ourselves. It is also true that people with eating disorders generally share a history of serious difficulty establishing who they are in relation to what they want and what others want from them.

Exploring our own strengths and limitations is a natural, lifelong process. One key prerequisite for enjoying that continuous personal development is the freedom to explore available choices and to compare those choices to personal interests and ideas. It will help if you think about your own life. For many people, the years before and during elementary school were fairly structured. Parents, teachers, and other adults defined the limits of your world. If they set clear rules about what was good or bad for you, you probably followed those rules, at least when they were watching.

If you were the kind of youngster who followed every rule, then you may have based your success or failure on the reactions you got from the adults who were important to you. You would know you were good in school if the teachers said so. If your parents told you they were proud, then you knew you were successful, whether the topic was school, sports, or socializing. If pleasing others was your primary means of knowing success, you were the most compliant child possible. You probably did not spend much time or thought on determining whether you had pleased yourself by your behavior. Your focus would basically have been on how other people rated your behavior.

If you focused all your energy and creativity on finding out how to play by the rules and then playing to achieve perfection, then every day of your life was like opening night at the theatre. Everyone important was watching, and your performance had to be flawless. If the critics felt you failed, your own feelings would be irrelevant. Your play would still be closed. So you had to keep the show going by finding out what the critics, the grown-ups, expected, and then giving them what they wanted every day. That way, you were guaranteed rave reviews. The applause was the message you needed to let you know you were still acceptable.

There was just one problem. The audience kept changing. First, there was just your mother and father. Maybe there were other family members, but your world did not reach much beyond family, an occasional neighbor, some other children, and the doctors who checked you up and helped your parents keep you healthy. All those people set the rules, and you followed them. The more you followed the rules, the happier they were, because when you followed those rules, they felt you were safe.

As you got older, more people got involved in making rules for you. There were schoolteachers and spiritual leaders. Maybe there were coaches or neighbors who played an important part in your life. No matter who they were, they had rules and expectations. If you were a compliant child who felt successful only if an adult said you were successful, then you perfected the art of understanding the rules and giving the performance of your life, every day of your life. Some people set the stage, others wrote your lines, still others prepared your costumes, and you delivered the performance precisely. Then you waited for the applause, the curtain went down, and you went to sleep, so you could do the whole thing again the next day.

The Cinderella Effect:
Creating Your Own Self-Image

Boys and girls who live every day like an opening night can find a kindred spirit in Cinderella. They feel trapped by their own emptiness and limitations, but they feel powerless to escape. Just as Cinderella slaved daily to please those around her, these youngsters work tirelessly to do the expected. They do not consider risking failure, punishment, and even outright rejection or abandonment by initiating such a bold action as taking on a new role.

Like Cinderella, these young people choose their role. Cinderella chose to accept the way she was treated, rather than resist the role her family gave her. She grew up preferring the predictable life her family defined for her, rather than risking the unknown and carving out a place for herself based on her own perception of herself.

The Fairy Godmother could only work her magic if Cinderella was willing. Cinderella had to believe that she could improve her life. As soon as she believed that she could really fulfill her own dream, she was successful. The Fairy Godmother gave the coach and the dazzling dress, but Cinderella had to accept the self-concept and pursue her dream. It was Cinderella who made the entrance, and Cinderella who made the impression. Her success was her own.

Many of us grew up thinking that Cinderella was rescued, first by the Fairy Godmother and then by the Prince. We ignored the simple and straightforward fact that Cinderella had to *decide* to go to the ball. She had to *choose* to risk ridicule and rejection by going up to the prince and presenting her foot, so he could see for himself that the shoe fit her and her alone.

Cinderella only needed one night as a princess to get the confidence necessary to create her own identity. She was able to see that her potential was her own, and that her identity was something she could invent and control. Far from being a weak, dependent character who always needed other people to define who she was, Cinderella became stronger and more assertive as soon as she discovered that she could be who and what she chose.

As you well know, Cinderella chose to give herself the best possible life she could create. Children who focus all their creativity and energy on creating an identity to please others often fail at the one lesson so important to growing up: Outside the world of make-believe and perfect, happy endings, each of us really can try on new faces and create our own special selves.

Inside fairy tales of desperate crisis and perfect endings, there are threads of truth grounded firmly in reality. It is true that children can find themselves utterly dependent on other people for every good or bad feeling they experience. And it is true that they can change that dependency gradually, over time, as they experiment with different options and ideas. Often, the catalyst that helps them see their own power and creativity is a trusted person whom they identify as a partner, committed to empowering them to grow and become more competent every day.

Cinderella spent her entire childhood and early youth focusing all her energy on maintaining the identity she accepted from the people who defined her world. As soon as she decided to step in and define some of her world on her own, she saw that she could also define her identity. The fact that she could do what other people wanted simply meant that she could also do what she wanted. From that point on, things could get better for her, with or without the Prince.

Like Cinderella, people who suffer from anorexia, bulimia, or bulimarexia often go through childhood identifying what other people expect and then living up to those expectations. They often adopt the identity that others have chosen for them, and they fulfill every expectation to the very best of their ability. Anything less than their very best causes them pain and suffering, as they doubt their own self-worth and invest everything in setting, accomplishing, and surpassing concrete goals. Then comes adolescence.

Self-Image and Adolescence:
The Connection Between
Eating Disorders and Puberty

When children work tirelessly to please adults, and navigate their preschool and elementary school years with great care to follow the rules, they can find adolescence more than disturbing, confusing, or unsettling. They can find it impossible. In trying to pinpoint when it became clear that life was changing without her consent or control, Evette DiMartino recalls sitting at the kitchen table with her parents, going over the school's course-options handbook available to youngsters entering seventh grade.

It was a typical scene—me and my parents sitting at the kitchen table, talking about schoolwork. But this time, I was in a panic. And I mean in a genuine panic. Think about the feeling you might get if you were stuck on a dark, lonely road, miles from home, in the middle of the night, and a carload of creeps stops right next to your car. They get out, and one of them has a gun. Unless you were armed and prepared for that to happen, you would probably get really scared. If you admit it, you'd probably panic. Well, it was the same for me. It seemed like everyone else was armed and prepared for all this new decision-making, except for me. And I couldn't believe it. I was always on top of everything.

You can't really blame me for being so confused. Every other year I'd ever been to school, I was told what teachers I would have and what subjects I would take. Now I had to choose when I would take certain courses, and even whether I would take those courses. Yes, I had to take all the basic subjects. But then I had to decide if I would take orchestra or chorus or both. I had to figure out if I wanted to take shop and then home economics, or home ec and then shop. And I had to pick a language: French, Spanish, Italian. I couldn't believe it. And I felt so strange inside. You may think this sounds crazy, but I could feel my body changing all the time. It was a new shape, and there were new things to worry about. Like boys.

I can honestly say my parents never pushed me to date before I was ready, or to do things that I said I didn't want to do. I just never really expressed any opinion, because I didn't really have an opinion. I was only interested in doing what they wanted me to do. I remember they sat with me, all concerned, and they said, "Honey, you've always been the perfect student. School is school. You'll be at the top of your class, as usual. Sure, your social life will start to change. You'll like boys and want to go out more. But you can do it. You always have! You're just growing up now, and you have to make some decisions on your own."

As soon as they said that, I heard this voice inside me say, "Hey! You can't do that! You can't abandon me now! How can you say 'just growing up'! This is really scary! How does a person grow up? What are the rules?" Of course, I didn't say that out loud. I didn't want to sound stupid, but I was very nervous, and really angry. Everything was different, and they were pretending that nothing important had really changed, except that I had a few new responsibilities, and I had to make sure I didn't take drugs or have sex before I was ready. That's what all the adults worried about. Meanwhile, I was worried about how to get through the first day of school. I figured, if I was worried about things they thought weren't important, then I must be bad at growing up. Sometimes I felt stupid, but mostly I felt crazy.

No matter where I went, I felt crazy. School, home, the park, church, bike-riding, softball—it didn't matter. Everything felt different, and I felt crazy. Even when I was all alone in my room at home, I felt crazy. All these different thoughts kept rushing through my head. It was like I couldn't control my own head! And my body—forget it. All of a sudden, it felt like people were looking at me and talking about me....I just felt

like running away as fast as I possibly could, but I [?]
was out. Kids who run away get killed or wors[?]
concentrated on getting things in order.

It's like being a teenager was a big surprise for me. I
know that everyone in my family used to tease about how
good I was, and how I would get over being so good once I
became a teenager. My parents and aunts and uncles
always fooled around about that stuff, but I didn't really
think about it. I figured that life would stay pretty much the
way it always had been. I never got into the stupid trouble
that other kids always got involved with, so—I figured that
if I stayed in control, doing the things I always did, I would
be okay.

Well, I was wrong. And my parents were wrong, too. School
is not the same throughout all the years. The whole thing
about making friends changes, teacher expectations change,
your social life changes—adolescence even changes the way
you think and deal with information and emotions. No one
told me that so much of it was out of my hands. I thought
that if I was strong enough and followed all the rules, I could
cope with being a teenager just the way I coped with everything else. But it's a whole lot more complicated than saying
no to drugs or making sure that you stay away from the kids
who are always in trouble.

Being a teenager is weird. Everyone jokes about it, and
parents make a big deal about drugs and sex, but I think kids
get in trouble with drugs and sex because they can't sort out
how they feel. It's so hard to figure it all out. All through the
first part of your life, everyone tells you what to do and when
to do it. Then you go through puberty, and all of a sudden
they start telling you that you're older now, as if you didn't
know, and that you have to start taking more responsibility for
your actions and decisions.

Well, no one in the world took more responsibility for their
actions than I did, for as long as I can remember. I felt I was
responsible for everything and for everyone's happiness.

When I succeeded at something, I did it for everyone, because I felt responsible for making them happy. But then the rules started to change, my body started to change—even my brain started to change. And there were so many more people I had to please. All those teachers, and new kids....Ugh. It was impossible.

No matter how much I hated it, or how much I wanted to just hide, I couldn't. You can't just drop out of everything. So I decided that if I was good enough, I would do everything. And I did. I went to my guidance counselor and told her I was confused. That's when I learned that your guidance counselor will tell you what to do if you act really confused and overwhelmed. Of course, I didn't have to act. She said, "No problem, honey!" and it was over. I had a schedule, and I had extracurricular stuff because my parents thought that was important. I had band and chorus, and I signed up for every sport that was in season. You know—track, swimming, that stuff. I loved that, because the coaches were great. They told you what to do, told you to try your best, and then they sat back and watched. So I got to learn the rules, try my best, and really impress the coach.

My coach in track was my regular gym teacher, and we got really friendly. She said that if I really committed myself to training, I could be Olympic material. I almost died! Me! An Olympic track star, standing up there with the gold medal around my neck...what a dream.

I told my parents, and they really got into it, too. It was great. I could spend all my free time training, and I could get a trainer. They would pay for it, and they would send me to camps to get the right training. I could fill up every minute with this new thing, and I could get applause as big as the United States! I was so excited I couldn't breathe. I started to run more and more, every day and every night. Some of the kids teased me, but who cared? I was shooting for the Olympics.

I remember going to a state meet, and all the girls from all over the place were in the same locker room. Everyone was really intense—it was like being in a room filled with me, everywhere I looked. That was the first time I remember really looking at other girls' bodies and seeing that they were trimmer than I was. Their muscles looked tighter and better developed, and they didn't have that skin that moved back and forth when they ran. I asked my coach about that, and she said that my thighs just had baby fat, and that the fat would go away if I trained more and cut down on the bad foods, like the sugar and fat. Right away, I told my parents. If they wanted me to make the Olympics, they had to help me diet. And they did. My mother cooked separate meals for me and helped me put together my good-food, bad-food list to stick on the refrigerator. I started to run in those tight, stretchy pants, so no one would see my thighs wiggle. And I started training even harder.

I was really proud. I figured out how to beat the adolescence thing, and I was beating the big weight problem. Think about it. Teenagers are always complaining about being bored, and they're always getting into some kind of trouble— hanging out with the wrong kids or fighting with their parents. I had it all figured out! And I never had to fight with my parents. If I got angry with them, I would push the feelings down, so we just didn't have any of those wide-open intense conflicts that parents always complain about when they talk about teenagers.

So I thought I had adolescence all figured out. And I thought I had the whole weight thing under control, too. And that really made me special. I mean, when people aren't talking about how they can't handle their parents or they can't handle their kids, they're talking about how they can't handle their weight. They laugh about it, or they bitch about it, but they all say the same thing—they just don't have the willpower to turn down all that food. Well, I had the willpower. I could train for competition, and I could turn down any food any time. I remember feeling like I was on a constant high.

And the pain? Sure, there was pain. It was incredible. Between the hunger and the muscle pain from the constant workouts? I can't tell you how much I hurt.

You may think I was crazy to put myself through constant, intense pain. But you have to remember. I was fighting a battle. And when you get hurt in a battle, you're proud of it. Sure, you may scream inside, but if you're brave and really good, then you take it quietly, because you know it's the price you pay for winning. And I needed to win. I really felt that if I didn't win, I would die. All the different pressures and choices and changes were so intense—it was like all these enemy troops were coming at me, and I had to outsmart them. If I could discipline myself enough—if I could keep myself lean and strong—then I could win. The pain was just a natural thing I had to deal with.

Today, when I look at pictures of myself in running clothes, I gasp, just like you would. I mean, I look like one of those famine victims. I didn't need an enemy to come and get me—I had myself. But you couldn't tell me anything back then. I remember my mother making me food, and my father saying the meals were good enough to tempt the Gods, but I didn't eat. I know that drove them crazy, but none of us actually fought about it. I remember overhearing my mother's friend asking my parents if they got angry at me, and my parents said, "Of course not! We don't get angry with each other in this house. And anyway, she's got special pressures on her, with all this Olympic training. How could we add to all that? All the athletes go through this kind of thing at one point or another."

They really got themselves to believe all that shit. That we didn't get angry, and that all the other competitors starved themselves. Christ. We were all so out of touch with reality. Until I had passed out on the track for the third time in four meets, and my coach pulled me out of competition.

If it was you or your kid, maybe you would have realized that you had to thank the coach and face up to the facts—

that the future Olympian wasn't going to make it through the big race of life if she didn't get her act together. Well, not me. And not my family. We all ganged up on the coach. Me, my mother, my father. We all blamed the coach for pushing me too hard, making me diet—no one ever looked me in the eye and said, "Evette, you have made yourself very sick. You have cost yourself a shot at the Olympics. Now you have two choices. You can live in pain and maybe die—or you can start dealing with the fact that you're human—and that means that you can't be perfect. If you're human, you have feelings, and you have to deal with those feelings, no matter what they are. You really have no choice, because the feelings are there. Even if you pretend they aren't. They're still there. So you can face them, understand them, and learn how to cope with them, or you can kill yourself pretending they aren't there."

Anyway, I wanted to keep running, even though the coach said I couldn't until I got back to my regular weight of 100 pounds. My parents agreed, and that was when I began to hide the running. I would pretend I was doing other things, and I would sneak in at least five miles a day. I managed to do that perfectly, until I passed out in the woods, and I cut my head on a stone. There was no way I could hide that cut, and when I got home, my parents went crazy. I mean, it was the first real fight I ever had with them in my whole life.

As soon as I walked in the door, everything hit the fan. First, they went bananas because I had this big cut on my head. They made me wash it, and then they made me go to bed. I have this huge four-poster bed, and I was lying on top of my bedspread, up against the stuffed animals and the pillows...My mother was sitting in the white rocker that's under the window...She was just rocking and crying. My father—God. He kept pacing back and forth and hollering—I don't remember what he was saying. I was just watching what he looked like when he was angry at me.

It was like someone else was lying in the bed, and I was outside the window, looking in, watching this girl make her parents furious. It had to be someone else, because I never got my parents angry enough for them to have a fight with me. I could not handle it. I couldn't cry, I couldn't answer them, I was just scared and amazed. Then my father said something about making me go away to some hospital where they would make me eat and exercise like a normal person.

You can bet I woke up then. This voice inside me said, "See! You were right! They find out that you're not perfect, and right away, they want to get rid of you!" I figured, this is war again—get it together or they really will send you away.

I begged, pleaded, and put on my most perfect Evette-the-good-little-girl act, and they finally said I could live at home if I would agree to go to a doctor. I agreed, because I figured one doctor would be easier to control than a whole hospital full of doctors. Well, I handled those doctors, the way I handled everyone else. I did what they wanted, impressed them with how good I was, and they would finally tell my parents that I was fine. I put on such a good show, they would end up thinking that I was fine, and my parents were the ones who needed the shrink. I was having a great time, because I was getting all these doctors to fight with my parents, and I didn't have to do anything but act perfect. It was great.

Anyway, we went to about six different types of doctors before my father found this thing in the paper about Dr. Zimmer. I figured, here we go again. I went, because I was good at going to doctors. But Dr. Zimmer was a whole different kind of person. He was really friendly, but he was very direct. He looked me right in the eye, and I knew that he knew exactly what I was doing to myself. He understood how crazy I felt. After a few months, I got up the courage to trust him a little, and I remember I said something about how much I hated being a teenager. He said he understood how much I must hate it, and I swear—I couldn't believe it. He didn't just laugh and tell me it was a phase. He didn't even make a joke, or ask me stupid questions about sex or boys or if I was afraid of dating. He did say something that totally blew my mind.

I can't remember the exact words, but—basically, he said that being a teenager meant feeling all sorts of things all at once, because your body and your emotions and even your brain start to go through all kinds of changes. He said that sometimes people try to deal with all those feelings by getting totally absorbed in something that helps them control their bodies and minds. Some kids use drugs or alcohol. Then he asked me what I thought I did to try to stay in control of those feelings, and I started to cry. I think I cried for an hour before I finally said that I starved myself. I finally said it out loud.

Evette was ashamed and afraid to admit that she starved herself. She preferred to hide under fashionable layers of oversized sweaters and big loose jackets. Her skirts were always very full, and if her pants were snug, then her sweaters or shirts or jackets hung far below her hips. She tried desperately to please her doctors, please her parents, look like any other teenager, and still succeed in hiding deep inside herself. The starving caused her constant, intense pain. But from Evette's point of view, the pain she inflicted on herself was tolerable, because she controlled it, and it was consistent.

All her life, Evette had found great comfort in establishing one way to react or feel, and then eliminating all the other possible feelings. She was a success—a lovable child who made everyone happy. Once she became a teenager, she began to have feelings she could not control. Those feelings ranged from wonderful to horrible, but they had two things in common: They were new, and they were strong. She had never felt this way before, and the turmoil she felt inside made her intensely anxious. That anxiety was physically and emotionally painful. The fact that she could not predict how or what to feel at any given time was simply unacceptable to her. After years of depending on her parents and teachers to help her know what to think and feel, she was simply unprepared to cope with all the physical, emotional, social, and academic changes that were part of being a teenager.

All around her, Evette saw change. Her friends were changing. Her school was changing. Her body was changing. Her parents seemed to think she was ready for that change, but her doubts were overwhelming. She had no frame of reference for solving problems by herself. Her parents told her it was time for her to learn—to grow up and make some decisions for herself. The implication was that anyone her age should be ready to take on new responsibilities. Since Evette knew that she was not ready, she felt she was a failure. She had spent virtually her entire life pleasing her parents, and they suddenly changed their expectations. She had always been able to live up to their standards, and she was terrified that she could not handle their new expectations.

Yes, Evette was angry that her parents let her be such a perfect little follower and then suddenly expected her to be the leader in her own life. But she could not risk letting them see her anger, because that may upset or disappoint them. Evette's solution was to find some territory to control, some rules to follow, and then show her parents how much she could achieve.

The territory she chose to control was her body. The rules she chose to follow were the rules of the long-distance runner. She soaked up direction—from diet books, coaches, teachers, friends, other athletes—anyone who could give her rules to follow so she could achieve concrete goals. Losing weight was a concrete goal. Keeping it off was a concrete goal. Pacing herself in a race was a concrete task. If it was concrete, then Evette could do it. Growing up was not concrete. It was vague and confusing, full of contradictions and feelings that could appear and disappear suddenly and violently. If Evette allowed those feelings to come and go—if she allowed herself to feel the way a teenager feels—she knew she would have to change. She knew it was impossible to please her parents, please all the new teachers, and still let herself feel what a regular teenager feels—confused, wonderful, rebellious, confident, and insecure, sometimes all at the same time.

Adolescence is unsettling for just about everyone. But youngsters like Evette have an especially hard time, because they have spent the early part of their lives struggling so hard to please other people. When they achieve something, they do not feel proud until a parent or another important adult tells them to feel proud. By the same token, if they achieve a goal, and an adult does not approve, then they will suppress any sense of pride or accomplishment and feel what the adult says is appropriate.

It's important for kids to know how adults feel, but the reverse is equally important. When kids grow up with a reasonable sense of confidence in their own feelings, then they are in a position to make choices on the understanding that some of their decisions will be good, and some will be bad. It's part of being human, and part of growing up. But when kids grow up depending on adults to let them know when and what to feel, adolescence can be impossible to manage, since being a teenager means spending more time with friends, more time with choices to make, and less time with adults nearby to tell you what is or is not okay.

Evette was just such a youngster, paralyzed by the range of choices, feelings, and pressures that came along with adolescence. After nearly a year of care, Evette has learned how to weigh and manage feelings, instead of food. She is still afraid to give up certain food rituals, but she is working on that fear. At the Biofeedback and Psychotherapy Center, Evette found a special combination of traditional counseling and independent self-control training in the form of biofeedback. When adults or teenagers like Evette become so desperate for a sense of control over their lives that they starve, binge, or purge, they may be able to take real control over the disorder through a special process called biofeedback. In the following chapter, you will discover what biofeedback can do for a teenager or an adult who suffers from anorexia, bulimia, or bulimarexia.

9 | Biofeedback: What Is It, and How Does It Help?

I went into therapy because I needed to answer to somebody. I stayed in therapy, and the doctor helped me learn how to answer to myself.

—Geri Erikson, age 34
Recovering bulimic

If you are bulimic, anorexic, or bulimarexic, you probably work extremely hard to control what happens to your body. Biofeedback is a very effective, rewarding way to monitor and eventually control different physiological processes, like your heart rate, muscle tension, and perspiration levels. If you can monitor the way your body reacts to different thoughts and tensions, then you can learn how to control your body's reaction to stress. If you binge, purge, or starve in order to cope with stressors that are dominant issues in your life, then biofeedback can be part of an overall treatment plan that can help you do the two things you want most: stay in control of your body, and get healthy.

When Geri Erikson finally came to the Biofeedback and

Psychotherapy Center, she had been bulimic for eleven years. She said she was willing to try a combination of stress management training, biofeedback, nutritional guidance, and psycho therapy so that she could be free of the disorder that had come to dominate her life.

I had gone for help twice before. First, I went to a woman who was helping a friend of mine. I told the woman that I really wanted to stop, and she told me to give up on that goal—that I would always do it. Then I went to another doctor, and he gave me sedatives to calm my nerves.

The third one I went to said that my eating problems were a clear sign of sexual guilt, and he asked me "Do you masturbate?" Can you believe that? I wasn't in his office ten minutes, and he said that. I had just finished telling him that two to five times every day of my life for eleven years, I had been eating pounds of food and then throwing it all up, because I was hooked on the feeling I got from vomiting. I told him that it made me feel like I was throwing up the world. And he asked me if I masturbate.

Needless to say, I left and didn't go back. I was ready to just give up, when a friend of mine told me that her sister was really happy going to Dr. Zimmer. I went, and I knew immediately that this was a person I could depend on to help me. I was really motivated to stop, but I already knew I couldn't do it on my own. It's like kicking alcohol. You really need support to help you through the crisis times.

You see, I always thought the whole bulimic thing was disgusting. On my thirteenth birthday, my 16-year-old brother told me that he could eat everything he wanted, because he would just throw it all up as soon as he was really full. I remember thinking, Ugh! How disgusting! But you know how it is when someone plants an idea in your head? Well, that's what happened with me. When I looked at my brother, he looked like he was in good shape. He even looked like he felt better because he did it. So I tried it, and I know it probably sounds sick, but it really did feel good.

Purging is a good word to describe what I did. I really purged myself of everything I hated in me and in everything else. It was a way of getting rid of every poisonous feeling I had, and it was so rewarding to be in charge of the whole process.

After a while, I really got involved in all kinds of food games and rituals, just to see how much I could control what I took in or eliminated from my body. I would fast for weeks, binge, purge, and go around and around like that, feeling totally cleansed.

Then one night, I nearly choked to death. I couldn't clear my air passage, and I nearly passed out in the basement, in the private corner where no one went, where I used to throw up into a plastic bag. I dropped the bag—Ugh. It was horrible. I got so scared that night, I decided to stop for a while.

I remember feeling so many different things—it was bizarre. Mostly, I was embarrassed, you know, because I wanted to go for help, but I didn't want anyone to know I was hooked on eating pounds of food and then throwing it up. I mean, it's a totally disgusting thing to do, and it's hard to think that anyone will like you or care about you if you admit that you do it.

I honestly believed that it would be impossible for me to lie to a doctor I respected and wanted to impress. Basically, I was looking for a new version of what my parents used to be. I wanted to find someone to please, and I would please them by following their rules, which would include eating normal amounts, not bingeing or purging or fasting.

Dr. Zimmer listened to this whole speech I made about needing someone to report to. He let me go through the whole speech I had rehearsed, and then he said we might be able to reach an agreement, but I had to be willing to bargain. He said I could keep the goal of taking control over the eating problems, but I would have to report to myself—not to him.

As soon as he said that, I got scared, way down in the bottom of my stomach. I told him I had never relied on myself to monitor or change my own behavior. You know what he said then? He said "You've been monitoring and changing your behavior for years, every time you decided to binge, purge, or starve. You decided to do something to achieve some kind of change in the way you felt."

What could I say? He was right. I just never looked at it that way. So he keyed in on my need to really control and know what was happening inside me, and he helped me learn how to do biofeedback, which is great. Basically, you use a biofeedback machine, which is sensitive to your heart rate, your sweat-gland activity, or other physical things that indicate how relaxed or stressed you are. At first it was frustrating, because I couldn't get anything to happen. I could interpret the signals the machine was giving, so I could monitor whatever physical dynamic I wanted to watch, like my heart rate. But it felt like it would take forever until I could really control my heartbeat.

Dr. Zimmer was really patient through the whole thing. He said it takes time to learn the process, and he showed me how to relax and get to know the machine. I was motivated to learn how to control the way my body reacted to stress, because I knew I would binge and purge anytime I would get this really anxious, intense feeling inside that wouldn't go away until I literally threw it up.

So, every week I would go to the doctor, and I would have a regular therapy session where we would talk, and then I would spend time at the biofeedback machine, getting to know what was going on in my body, and learning how to control different things going on inside me. Now that I've learned how to use the machine better, it makes me feel so powerful. More powerful than I felt when I was bingeing and purging, because I don't feel ashamed. I feel proud. And I know that if I have a bad day, it isn't going to be bad for the whole rest of my life. I used to panic if anything went wrong at home, in school, at work—if I wasn't doing everything right, I felt like I was doing everything wrong.

It's been eight months and three days since my last bulimic episode. I feel so proud of myself. I really do. The doctor keeps telling me that the accomplishment is my own, and I do believe him, most of the time. You know, it's strange that we're talking today, because it was exactly a year ago this weekend that I tried to kill myself. There had been a big blow-up in my family—my sister-in-law, Lynn, had really been obnoxious to my mother, so I called Lynn up and told her that she really shouldn't talk to my mother like that. I did it because my mother was so upset, ranting and raving about how Lynn hurt her, and how she gets heart palpitations every time Lynn talks to her—I was afraid my mother would have a heart attack if this kept up! So as soon as my mother heard me tell Lynn to try to be a civil human being to my mother, my mother grabbed the phone and yelled at me for butting in.

I can't tell you how desperate I got at that moment. I felt that I was totally helpless and useless. My mother preferred that piece of garbage Lynn to me, her daughter. I could never do anything right, and I was always trying so damn hard. At that moment, everything went black. It was as if I had a total eclipse inside my head, and a giant, painful mass blocked out every bit of life I had in me. I couldn't feel anything. I just went into the bathroom, locked the door, smashed the mirror on the medicine cabinet, took a piece of glass, and hacked at my wrists until I passed out.

They tell me I was on the floor 15 or 20 minutes before they finally got in the bathroom. They called an ambulance and all, and I was pretty surprised that they were so upset. I really thought they wouldn't notice if I was there or not.

Anyway, just after that whole crisis, I read the story about how Jane Fonda had the same sickness I did. I was amazed. I really think she did a public service, letting people know that someone as perfect as she looks is really just another human being. I talked about this with Dr. Zimmer, and while we were talking, I started to cry and laugh at the same time. I suddenly realized that if Jane Fonda—who was so beautiful and successful—couldn't be perfect, then I couldn't be perfect, either. It was finally okay to just be human!

That may be obvious to you, but it took me months of using that biofeedback machine and working through feelings in the regular sessions with Dr. Zimmer before I finally figured out that I could have human standards for myself and still be successful.

Now I keep coming so I can improve my skills with the biofeedback. I've learned so much about how to monitor my feelings and get rid of tension before it takes over my body....So I still see Dr. Zimmer for the therapy and the biofeedback, because successful recovery has its costs and painful stages, too. My best friend, who is also bulimic, told me I didn't need a doctor. She said she'd been bulimic for years, and if you ever saw her, you'd really think she read a book about how to look like the perfect American princess. I mean, she has it all—gorgeous house, perfect figure, rich husband. She had trouble conceiving for a while, and when I told her I thought it had something to do with her bulimia, she told me I was wrong.

She's pregnant now, and I think she's still actively bulimic. She denies it, but I don't believe her. Actually, she doesn't see me much anymore. It's as if she resents me for getting help. So sometimes helping yourself hurts. But not helping hurts more. I'm grateful I found Dr. Zimmer, and I'm really grateful that he didn't offer me magical cures or try to take over my recovery. I know I'm not well yet, but I am getting better, thanks to the biofeedback and regular therapy sessions.

I just want to add one thing. People should be afraid of this disorder. It can kill you. It can take over your life, and it can take your life. Biofeedback and psychotherapy worked for me. Maybe other people prefer support groups, more group therapy, or a combination of different treatments. The point is, the right kind of help is out there for you. You just have to go get it. You aren't the only one who has the problem. You aren't the only one who thinks it would be better to die than reveal everything to a doctor. I felt exactly the same way. But I knew, when I was lying on the basement floor and gasping for breath, that I didn't want to die like Karen Carpenter. I wanted to live. Living meant changing, and I know I'm here today because I chose life.

Choosing life means getting help. You might choose biofeedback or individual psychotherapy, or you may choose support groups or family, marital, or group therapy. If you have an eating disorder, you can find help that gives you the information, confidence, and insight you'll need to better understand and defeat the disorder. A treatment approach combining biofeedback and psychotherapy is just one method that can help you better understand and control your feelings, so you do not have to violently assault your body by bingeing, purging, or starving.

10 | Coming Back From the Brink: Leslie's Diary of Hospital Care

Sometimes, people who are bulimic, anorexic, or bulimarexic are simply too sick to go for help on their own. It may be very difficult for them to truly focus on changing while they are still living at home, or living in the place where they became ill. Or they may go to the doctor and pretend to change. After a while, the pretense will show. The weight may drop too far, or there could be medical problems that develop from bingeing and purging.

When treatment does not seem to be helping a person while he or she still lives at home and goes to school or work as usual, a special hospital program may be the best treatment choice. Some bulimic or anorexic people need the structure of a good hospital program so that they can stabilize physically and emotionally. Once they achieve that basic stability, it's possible for them to discover how they really can fit into day-to-day life, just the way Leslie Doyle came back to her home and school, after a hospital stay that saved her life.

"Watch Out, World! Leslie's Back and Better Than Ever!"

Leslie Doyle was hospitalized in February of her senior year in high school. She was five feet, eight inches tall, and on the day she entered the hospital, she weighed 89 pounds. The letters she wrote to her doctor became a shared diary that helped them both understand what the hospital experience was doing for her on a very personal level. Leslie agreed to share some of those letters with you, so you could understand how she felt when she was hospitalized, how she changed while she was in the hospital, and how being in that program helped her maintain her healthy new habits when she got back home.

Her first letter was full of the pain and shock of actually being hospitalized. She wrote how strange it felt to ride in her parents' car and look out the back window, watching her world recede as she was propelled into a strange new universe where she would stay long after her parents left for home.

For days before she actually left for the hospital, she planned how she might escape. Then she would feel guilty—guilty and angry at herself for letting her sickness get so bad that it was out of control. She had agreed not to lose any more weight, and she knew that if she lost even one pound, she would be put into the hospital. And she kept on losing weight. One side of her knew she had forced the doctor and her parents to hospitalize her. But the other voice inside her kept saying, "You'll beat this. Just do what they want really fast and get out, because they'll make you fat and disgusting, after you've worked so hard to get this thin."

With the voice inside her talking a mile a minute, the ride seemed to go by in a flash. The hospital was one of those huge old brick institutions with floor-to-ceiling windows and a wide, graceful flight of steps leading up to two big wooden doors. It looked as if it had been a private estate. Inside, it was a lot more like a hospital. Even though the ceilings were high and the molding was fancy, everything had an institutional feeling about it. There really were people in white coats who took everything from her the minute she went in. They emptied her pocketbook in front of her, took an inventory of the contents, and put anything they thought was dangerous into a big envelope for safekeeping.

After the basic admitting procedures were finished, Leslie watched her parents leave. Inside, she felt abandoned, desperate, angry, hurt, and scared to death. But she kept absolutely silent as the doctors, nurses, and assistants gave her a complete physical, took blood for tests, brought her to her room, and introduced her to her roommate, Carrie. She and Carrie became friends right away.

After she settled in, Leslie decided that the best way to share what she was living was to describe her day from the moment she woke up to the moment she went to bed. Of all the letters that we could choose from, Leslie felt you would best understand hospitalization as she experienced it if you could share this one letter she wrote just a few weeks after she was admitted.

March 15, 1986

Dear Dr. Sacker,

Hello! Today I'm going to do something cruel. Are you ready? You're going to spend the day with me here. It's Monday, 3/15/86, and it's 6:45 a.m. I was up at 6:30, but I decided to let you sleep a little longer. I thought you could get an idea of what it's like here. Today might be pretty busy, because it's Monday.

OK. We're in my room right now. I'm sitting at my desk and I can see out the window. It is a fabulous day—warm and sunny. From my window, we can see the tennis courts and two old-fashioned buildings that look more like large houses.

All right. Now it's 6:55 and I'm going to take you out into the hall. Come on! We're going to the restricted hall area, which consists of 2 sofas and a chair for the supervisor. Four girls are already out here with us, even though it's still dark.... We don't get weighed until 7:30, but it helps to get here early so we get a good spot in line. But of course, everyone cuts in front of me anyway. I'm new, and I don't really have a regular place in line. I also don't really care, I guess.

I have a sneaky feeling that Monday is the day they draw blood, so get ready. I can't stand it, myself. Last week I had a blood test in front of the other girls, and I cried. I was so embarrassed.

OK, the blood woman is here. It's 7:20 and Kim rushed to get her blood drawn first. Such eagerness. When Kim walks you can feel it on the Richter scale. She stomps on the floor and if she stands still she kicks anything in sight for about 10 minutes, and then she moves on to kick something else. One time it was the chair I was sitting in.

OH NO! When we go up to the blood woman we have to say our name. I can't talk in the morning. I'm really nervous. I'm glad you're here with me. Oh-oh—my turn.

OK, it's 7:30, and it's over. I kept myself to a near hiss noise. I will never forget the times you stayed with me when I was in the hospital in Brooklyn. You made the blood tests bearable. You helped today, too, so—thanks!

Here comes Merry, the head nurse. She's in charge of weighing us. She's really tough. SO NO HANKY PANKY. It's 7:40, and we've gone down through the far end of the hall, and we're in the Annex where all of Team A Eating Disorders gets weighed. I think everyone is in her own world at this time, and the tension is really strong. It's weird because, as I talk to you, I can step outside myself and see what this really looks like. There's Beth. I think I told you about her. She's the one who's been sick for 11 years. Anyway, she is pacing back and forth. She takes a step, waits two seconds, and takes another step. I'm positive she counts in her head. And she has to be weighed second. If she isn't second she gets hysterical.

Another girl, Mandy, does crossword puzzles while she waits. Dawn sits on the floor and curses to herself. Someone is jingling a watch, another reads, someone else fidgets, and still another one sleeps. I usually huddle in my robe and shiver as the chills go up and down my body.

7:50!!! My Turn!!

It's been rush, rush, rush ever since we stepped off the scale, so now it's 8:30. Anyway, Merry weighed me and somehow I went from 111 to 110 pounds. On Sustical, no less. [Sustical is a high-calorie nutritious drink that helps bring the body back into some level of balance as the dangerously underweight person starts to gain.] Merry didn't look too merry. She then takes my blood pressure and pulse lying down and standing.

That Dutch woman from down the hall just said she can't understand how I wanted to be this thin because I am attractive and have the potential to be striking! I'm grossed out! And it's not like I'm thin. I'm already 110 pounds. I look like a tub of lard! LARDO, LARDO! I know. You don't want to "argue" with my "bad" voice. Oh, yeah, on Friday was the first time I cried in front of everyone, aside from blood tests. I was so overwhelmed.

They won't tell me my target weight for another 2 weeks, so you can imagine how I'm freaking out. Every day I picture it being 100 pounds more than the day before. I'm drinking Sustical and gaining to a goal I don't even know. What if my knuckles disappear? It's hard to give up all the bones. For a long time, they gave me strength.

Anyway.........

At 7:55 I rushed down the hall to get someone to

Supervise My Shower,
So You Have to Wait Outside!

We're forbidden to take showers after a meal, so...I had to get it in before breakfast. At 8:20, when breakfast was supposed to be served I rushed through my shower, while you were standing out in the hall. I managed to dress, wash, and do my room in 10 minutes.

At 8:10 a.m. we went into the dining room. The room that gives me an ulcer. I sit at the Sustical table. There are three of us on Sustical. I have 320 cc of Sustical and 160 cc of juice 6 times a day. Anyway. Mandy drinks with her mouth stretched into a smile. I can understand it if she doesn't want to touch the stuff to her lips, but that's not the case with her, because she insists on licking the container. GROSS. Then there's Sharon, who has the "It's not fair" argument with anyone and everyone. Don't let her get you down. I don't feel bad for her because it's her own fault that she's on Sustical. She reached her target weight, so it's not like she has to gain 30 pounds. If she ate everything on her tray, she would maintain weight.

9:30: Commodes (That's Toilets,
and It's Supervised)

9:35: I'm back. Are you grossed out or what? I go wild about having to clean up after it, but—at least it's over.

Anyway, back to what I was saying. I figured that eating makes Sharon freak out, but she's been caught sneaking food. OK, so you're right. She just likes to be obstinate, so people will fight with her. Mandy sneaks food also, so between the two of them they're making me insane. Plus, they always fight with each other. I have to admit, I have my own fetishes, but at least I don't argue...anymore....

Meanwhile, there is a staff member who sits right in front of us through mealtime, so we finish every drop. That's weird, in and of itself. Then you have the people on trays—that means they're new at eating real food—and they make me dread eating. To top it off, Team B people, who have absolutely no problem eating, complain all the time about the way we eat.

OK, so the dining room is not a country club. It's 9:45, and I've been sitting in the same spot on the sofa since 8:30 a.m. You must be thrilled so far. The kids who have school just left. I can't wait to start.

Break Time for Therapy!

11:30: I had a "one-to-one" with Theresa. She's my mental health worker, and she's the one who works specifically with my care plan. Everyone has a mental health worker, and everyone has a nurse. My nurse is Louise.

Anyway, she—I mean she and I—talked about rejection. She says I use vivid expressions to get my point across and that I am full of energy. Now she wants to see me use some of my energy more constructively. I told her it's impossible for me to talk with more than one person at a time without feeling like I'm facing a firing line, or performing for an audience.

I guess I don't think I'm good enough for a large group to accept or like me. Maybe I think two people is a large group. Anyway, Merry, the head nurse, said I was one of the few patients she liked very much, right from the beginning. So I told Theresa that I had a hard time understanding that someone could like me, just like that, without me even doing anything. So we set a goal.

MY NEW LONG-TERM GOAL:
I WILL ACCEPT MYSELF MORE,
AND LEARN TO BE MORE SOCIAL
AND COMFORTABLE IN SOCIAL SITUATIONS.
MY SHORT-TERM GOAL:
TO START A CONVERSATION WITH AT LEAST
ONE PERSON BY NEXT WEDNESDAY.
FREAK OUT TIME!!!!

After therapy, I went to restricted activities—that's an activity for anyone who isn't allowed to do anything. I'm new, so I'm not allowed to do anything. So the restricted activity is art. I'm making a T-shirt.

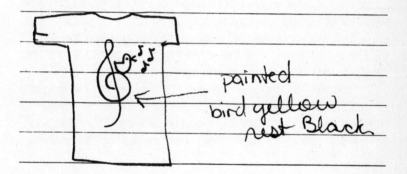

painted
bird yellow
nest Black

Since there wasn't any black paint, I made an Easter card for my parents. Easter is next Sunday.

11:30 Was Commodes Again (Remember? Toilets.)

And now I'm waiting for Sustical and juice. The school kids came back just in time for lunch.

12:16: Lunch!!! Sustical and Juice

OK. It's 12:45 now. I just can't stand it—the whole eating situation really upsets me. I don't mind the drinking—well, that's not true, I do mind. But it's better than having to eat to gain the weight. Still, it bothers me. I think I'll finish my Easter card. Come on! Let's go!

How in! A woman here has a videotape of herself on the Jackie Gleason show. She was only 12 years old, and she's singing with her two sisters. Wow!

:)

Well, it's 2:30 now. We had Sustical at 2:00. I played a game with Janet, who's going through all kinds of changes. See, she's bulimic, and she isn't really underweight like the rest of us, but she does a lot of the same things we do. It's weird. She really is very nice, and we get along great.

Tomorrow I'll be interviewed by a panel of doctors about nothing else but eating. And guess what! Tomorrow I'll have my school interview! Hooray! Maybe I can start soon. I'm really going to work hard and make up for previous stuff....

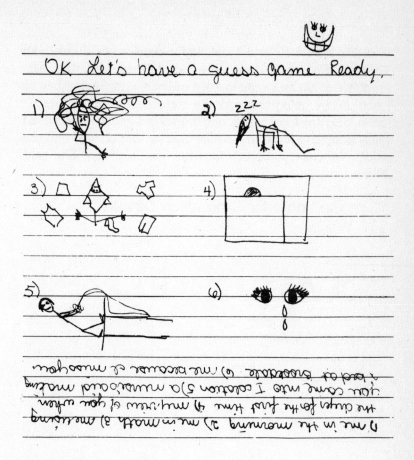

OK Let's have a guess game Ready.

1) 2) z²z

3) 4)

5) 6)

1) me in the morning 3) me in mud 8) me taking the chutes for the first time 4) me mirror of you when you come into 5) a musical and making food or breakfast 6) me because of moochou

Well, it's now 4:10 and I just had a session, or a talk, with Theresa. So anyway, we were just talking, and then she mentioned that they want to keep me here until September, so I wouldn't be going home for the summer. Of course, I wasn't thrilled. So anyway, I mentioned the school interview, and that I really wanted to finish my regular course work on time and she said... Wait, are you ready for what she said? Yes? She said

I Can Go Home for Graduation Day!!!!!!

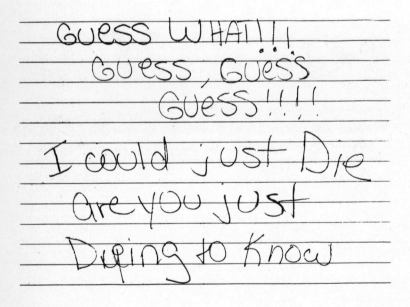

GUESS WHAT!!!
GUESS, GUESS
GUESS!!!!!
I could just Die
are you just
Dying to Know

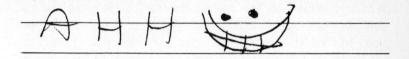

I'm Having Heart Palpitations With Happiness!!!!!

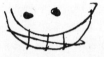

Of course, this is all based on my cooperation, but they say that so far, I've been doing beautifully, and I'm winning the staff's hearts.... Ahhhh.... It must be a gift. So I can go home for graduation if I do okay. I just know I can do it! Tell me, are you thrilled? I just knew you would be. Thanks.

I really think the staff likes me because I went through my Obnoxious stage at Brookdale. It's hard for me to believe that was me....

OK. Now it's 5:10 and dinner is in 5 minutes. I'm still happy. Janet has worked out her strangeness and has figured out that she can really make it here, just as I did. I'm glad she's staying.

Observation of the day: Team B has a new admission, and it's a male.

Are you ready? Dinner for me is Sustical, of course, but the others are having Salisbury steak and mashed potatoes and there's a scandal because it's all what they call "institutional food." Can you believe it? Who cares?

5:15: Dinner. Need I say more?

Now it's 5:45, and we're in the living room watching "What's Happening." There's a girl here named Sally—she's from Team B and she's the blonde on the other side of the room. She changes clothes 4 times a day and washes clothes 2 times a day. Weird.

Now it's 7:00 p.m. At 6:30 I went to exercise group for people confined to the unit, and now I'm genuinely ill. It's really an easy class, but I'm still weak, and my bones just grind into the floor. The staff is now "concerned," so I have to cut down on the exercise. But it's really good to have those exercise classes because it makes gaining weight a little less scary. The class only meets once a week. I hope I feel better next time I go. They're making me wait until next week.

Today is my day to call my parents, so maybe I'll do that now....

OK. Now it's 8:20, and I just got off the phone with my parents. Last time I called I was thrilled, but this time I'm just feeling jumpy and weird. I don't know. It was just strange, like they don't know what to say. I think they think I don't want to talk about being here. I don't know.

8:30: Sustical!

OK, now it's 9:45, and we're watching the Academy Awards with 7 other girls. Alan Alda is host, along with Jane Fonda. Isn't Alan Alda just a terrific actor? I think I've been living in a cave this year. I haven't seen any of these movies. OKAY! OKAY! I know I was living in a cave! I just can't believe I missed so much life.

Anyway, it's 10:30 now, and we're back in my room, commodes washed, faces cleaned, and teeth brushed. I just made my bed and it's just perfect. I learned how to do those tight sheets from Miss Alan at Brookdale. She made the best beds. Here, we have to make our own. It's really dark out and it's another day tomorrow. Thanks for spending the day. We better get some sleep.

Good night.
You're the best.

Love, Leslie

On May 12, Leslie wrote to say she was continuing to gain weight but she was panicked.

Dear Dr. Sacker,

First things first. First, I'm very sorry I haven't written in a long time. I'm really having a rough time. If feeling awful happens just before getting better, I'm definitely on the road to recovery. On 4/23 I was very excited because I got new freedoms and unsupervised showers. But on 4/26, the whole fiasco started for me. That weekend I cried hysterically for hours. The staff tried to talk with me, but nothing helped. I felt like I was doing everything wrong—that I managed to be a major screw-up, even in a hospital where you have to be a real idiot to screw up. No one else agreed, so about 5 people called me "ridiculous," which didn't help.

On 4/29 everything just crashed. I was still feeling sick, so I refused 3 Sustical feedings and missed school. Then I had another session with Theresa. She took me out for a 40-minute walk, and we discussed my uncle situation—you know. My uncle, the disgusting, dirty old man. Theresa said we would have to tell my parents, and I just said "Oh" but I was freaking out. Before nightfall I was in a total panic. Looking back now, it really seems scary. All I wanted to do was kill myself any way I could. I was becoming impossible. Once they saw my bloody fingernails from ripping up my arms, they started to supervise every move I made. Needless to say, I couldn't sleep all night. I was sort of in a daze. Having the door wide open with that woman watching me didn't help. I just wanted to disappear— the same as when my uncle used to watch me and sneak up on me, even when everyone was home. . . . It was too much to even be alive, and the night felt like a death sentence that the executioner kept screwing up.

Very often, recovery means going back over some very painful territory. Leslie thought that she would be able to go through her entire hospital treatment without ever having to face the haunting anger and helplessness that had driven her deep inside herself years before. She was wrong. No one with bulimia or anorexia finds healing neat, orderly, or predictable. It can be wonderful, illuminating, painful, and scary. But most of all, it's personal, unique, and full of hope. It was the hope she had already developed that pulled Leslie through the abject terror she felt as her counselor helped her face her own private monster.

Since each and every anorexic and bulimic person is unique, it's impossible to say that any one single event or situation can always cause a person to develop an eating disorder. In Leslie's case, there was a chronic condition that sent her deep inside herself on a difficult, painful, and fruitless search for safety. Leslie needed to find safety in a make-believe world inside her own pain, because her uncle had begun to sexually abuse her.

Leslie was a victim of her uncle's sexual abuse for more than 6 years. Over those years, her uncle would regularly babysit for her, take her shopping, cook dinner with her, and spend time alone with her, and together with the rest of the family. At every opportunity, he would approach her, touch her, whisper things that would frighten her, and would threaten to tell her parents and her friends that she was dirty and bad with him when no one was looking.

She had tried to tell her parents, but she could not find the words. She tried desperately not to be left alone with him, but her parents were impatient with her protests and reminded her she was lucky to have someone who loved her to take care of her, when so many other children had to stay with strangers who could hurt them. Deep in her heart, Leslie yearned for a stranger. She thought that she could tell on a stranger and get her parents' support, but that she could never tell on her uncle without getting blamed.

Many victims of child abuse believe that they are responsible for being hurt physically, sexually, and emotionally. When the abuser is a close friend or family member, the victim's confusion, anger, frustration, and helplessness can be even greater than when the abuser is a stranger, since the child believes his or her parents will just get angry at the child for saying such things about someone the parents love, respect, and trust. The child often anticipates that Mom or Dad will say that the story is untrue and will deliver some sort of punishment that will just make a difficult life even worse.

The vicious cycle of fear, abuse, and fear of reporting can drive the child farther inside a private world of suffering, anger, loss of power, and deeply felt self-doubt. For Leslie, a combination of those factors contributed to her illness. Since the problems were there on her way into anorexia, she had to face them on her way out. Otherwise, they would continue to haunt her. She could not recover if she continued to deny and avoid the fact that she had been victimized by a man who was loved and respected by so many people. She had to face that reality or risk becoming even more gravely ill.

With help from her hospital counselor and her regular doctor, Leslie became strong enough to admit to herself that her uncle was sick and needed help that she could not provide. She faced the liberating truth that she was a victim, and that she did not deserve or ask to be hurt. Then, with all the support she required, she was able to tell her parents that her mother's brother had sexually abused her. Months after that initial confrontation, her mother faced a reality that she had long suppressed—that she had also been sexually abused by her brother, so many years ago that she had blocked the horror from her memory, much the way victims of other types of crime, violence, or trauma will suppress the memory of the incident deep in their subconscious mind.

While Leslie had the feeling that everything was crashing in on her, she was actually going through a normal stage in the process of recovery. Even though it felt like she was sliding backward really fast, she was still on an upward trend. She had enough resourcefulness, self-respect, and love for herself to listen—to let people who cared about her really express their concern and give her direction. All those positive feelings and messages about life eventually won out over the voice inside her that encouraged her to self-destruct, but not without a long and bitter fight for her life.

So, after a night like that, you know they wouldn't just let me go about my business like nothing happened. In the morning, a woman watched me go to the bathroom, weighed me (I lost a pound) and made me sit on a couch in my nightgown. At 9:00 a.m. I was allowed to get dressed and go to eating disorder group. I stayed behind a chair and didn't say a word, but it helped when some of the girls offered to help. Merry hugged me, and Theresa and I had another session. I begged to get off supervision, at least at the commode. I was desperate. So they put me on structured days like I had in the beginning, but she allowed me to go to school.

That night, I scratched myself up with a nail file, and the night after that I scratched myself with my nails. Over the weekend, I cut 6-inch sections in my arms with a safety pin, and I refused to talk to anyone about it. On Monday, the scratching stopped, and I promised to be good. Lucky for me my promises are still worth something because on Tuesday, the team gave me a second chance—so I got back unsupervised showers and regular food, plus courtyard privileges, which means sitting in a fenced-off area outside for 15 minutes. So far, I've kept my head and I plan never to do that much damage again. But I can feel all the weirdness inside, anyway. I constantly shake, and my blood pressure's gone from 110/80 to 150/90, which is still a lot better than the old blood pressure. Remember when it was 80/50?

Guess What!!!! It's Now Monday, and I Have Reached Target Weight!!!!!!!!

Finally! I have gained a grand total of 41 pounds. I look very different, but some of the girls told me I still look thin. I guess I should take their word for it. I ate food this morning after a 7 week liquid diet, and it was scary, but rumor has it that it gets better. Oh, well. I can't wait to leave and get on with things, but there are a few things I still have to "take care of," as they say here. How did I get into this mess?

Anyway, they'll let me have the highest level of freedoms here so long as I maintain my weight, so I'm trying hard. I want to go to graduation.

I hope everything is going OK for you. I think about you a lot, and that's because I really miss you and your weird ties (hee hee!).

Bye for now,
Lots of love from

Leslie

Finally—normal weight and ready for life!!

Coming Home

When graduation day arrived in her home town, Leslie was there. She was allowed home on pass for two days, after having been on complete free foods for a week. One month later, she was home for good.

Over the past several months, Leslie has been able to maintain her weight, even as she entered a nearby college part-time. She was able to work with Theresa to face her parents and let them know the secret that Leslie had kept locked inside her—that her uncle had molested her for years, and that she had been terrified to tell anyone.

Theresa and Leslie rehearsed that meeting with her parents. They talked about how they would approach the issue, and they role-played. When Theresa portrayed her parents, she would present them as silent or distracted, preferring to ignore the reality presented by their child. With Theresa's help, Leslie was able to present the truth to her parents, and her parents responded with stunned silence. It took them time in the session to absorb this new information, and Theresa was there for all of them—parents and child.

In the months that have followed, Leslie has finally begun to get her parents' support, recognition, and respect. Her parents have learned how to recognize her as more than a good little girl, and she has learned to expect more than approval from the other adults who are important in her life.

You could say that Leslie has come back to us from the brink of her grave. For her, hospitalization was the only choice. She needed structure and separation from family and everyone she knew, so she could begin the slow, delicate, painful process of recovery. It was impossible for her to remain at home and receive direct care only in weekly office visits. She simply needed to know that someone was always there to protect her from herself, her parents, her uncle and all the schoolmates and teachers whose affection and respect she simply could not accept.

Leslie remains in treatment as she continues to learn how to transfer the lessons she learned in the hospital into lessons that apply in her daily life. The day she left the hospital, she mailed one last letter, full of hopes and plans, and signed simply: WATCH OUT, WORLD! LESLIE'S BACK AND BETTER THAN EVER!

Those of us lucky enough to know Leslie agree whole-heartedly.

Maybe you remember how Leslie observed that watching the Academy Awards made her feel like she'd been living in a cave, because it had been more than a year since she had seen a new movie. When she made that point, she was describing just a little bit of life on the other side—the inside world of starvation. Starving required all her concentration and energy. So even though she accomplished a great many things as she went through each day, she could not remember them clearly.

Leslie accomplished things only so that she could get to the next task. She never allowed herself the simple pleasure of completing a task, feeling proud of her accomplishment, spending time with friends, or going to a movie. She just kept moving as fast as possible through every day, isolating herself as dramatically and rigidly as she was ultimately isolated in the hospital.

As Leslie says now, "Getting locked up ended up making me free." The same may or may not be true for others. Each anorexic, bulimic, or bulimarexic person is unique, needing different types of support. Hospital care is just one resource that can be there for you when you need it.

11 | Treatment and Recovery: The Two Go Hand in Hand

Anorexia, bulimia, and bulimarexia are disorders that respond to good, consistent treatment. Since each individual and family affected is different, treatment needs can vary widely. If you or someone you love is struggling to cope with an eating disorder, you will find it the most rewarding if you search for the kind of treatment that fits your needs *and* helps you learn to rely on yourself and others for strength, support, and love.

Whether you look for the right care in private or family therapy, a support group, biofeedback, a hospital program, or a combination of some or all of these, you can be sure that you can find a treatment approach that can help you or someone you care about to understand and defeat anorexia, bulimia, or bulimarexia. No matter what type of treatment alternatives you find helpful, it's crucial to understand that treatment is not necessarily cure.

Today, it's hard for me to believe that I was ever really so sick. But on other days, I feel like I'm less than an inch away from sliding back to the other side, deep into the comfort of isolation. I call them my reminder days, because I know they're a regular part of recovery for lots of people like me. So I keep going to the doctor. I don't go as often now, but I increase the visits if I feel shaky. I also joined a support group, which I really love. Those people are phenomenal. They really understand!

—Mary Anne Lieb
Recovering anorexic

For many people who become bulimic or anorexic, recovery is a lifelong process of learning to express and cope with their feelings in ways that do not involve food abuse or other types of self-destructive behavior. One of the most important things to keep in mind when you enter into any therapeutic program for the treatment of eating disorders is that you have to set realistic goals.

For example, you may decide that you deserve to get the help you need, so you pick up the telephone and call a number of different organizations or private practitioners specializing in the care of people with eating disorders. Telling a friend or loved one that you are really going for the care you deserve can help give you the structure and encouragement you may need to keep the appointment.

When you take those first steps, you may be full of hope and excitement that you will finally be able to leave the disorder behind and start living again. A word of caution, though: Even if you have been bingeing, purging, or starving for months or years, you may expect that the therapy will quickly give you the skills and strength to get back the control you used to have over your body and your eating. That kind of thinking is a setup for disappointment and discouragement.

It took time for you or the person you care about to become ill, so it will naturally take time to get in touch with the feelings that allowed the disorder to develop. It will take time to learn how to eat moderate amounts of good food. Anorexic people can become less fearful of fat. Bulimic people can learn how to moderate the size of a portion of food and then allow the food to digest despite every physical and emotional urge to expel it. But it all takes time.

Time is a critical aspect of treatment, no matter what type of care is involved. That means that bulimic and anorexic people can slip back after making considerable progress. *That's okay.* You just want to keep the slip in perspective, understand what happened, and keep on moving forward. It's liberating to discover that you are not perfect, and that you do not have to be perfect. No one heals without a struggle. No one just decides to get well and then never has another symptom or difficulty.

Recovery naturally includes rough periods, but the process is rewarding if you understand that the therapist cannot really "make you well" if you binge, purge, or starve. The therapist cannot simply make your family interact better and love one another in a way that makes everyone in the family feel strong and confident. Your psychotherapist, medical doctor, group leader, or support group network can help you understand the disorder and the treatment process. However, if you are in treatment, then you are in charge of what develops from that care.

No doctor can simply "make you well." Treatment for anorexia and bulimia is a discovery process, involving a partnership between the doctor or therapist and the person who has bulimia or anorexia. As Leslie's own letters to her doctor prove, even hospital care puts demands on the patient to participate in healing. As Leslie stabilized physically, she was able to put more energy into understanding how she became so ill and how she could protect herself from such self-destruction in the future.

The key word is future. The people you have read about here know that they have a future, and it's marked by hope. They have learned that recovery is possible, because they looked for and found care that empowered them to use their own resources and develop new ones on the way to recovery. They came to terms with the reality that they would recover a little bit at a time, and that it was okay to set short-term, real-life goals. They also learned to accept that being human means falling short of some goals sometimes.

The right care will help you accept that one slip does not have to mean a total crash. If you fall, you can pick yourself up again. Eating one cookie is not the same as eating a whole box. Bingeing and purging once in a week is not the same as bingeing and purging once every day. Losing five pounds when your health requires that you gain at least ten can be a signal, but it is not the same as losing twenty pounds.

Finding and working through a solid treatment process has helped many people learn how to recognize danger signals and gain control over their eating problems. In the process, they learned how to feel good about other things and other people outside themselves, their pain, and food. Along the way, they found family, friends, and teachers who encouraged them and believed in them, even when life appeared the most frightening choice of all.

IV

FOR PARENTS, TEACHERS, AND FRIENDS: WHAT YOU DO CAN REALLY HELP

12 | "You Aren't All Alone": A Message From Parents to Parents

When I was growing up, I never heard of anorexia. When my son started to make lists of good foods and bad foods, I just figured he was dieting. Everybody diets. And he was successful. But who ever heard of starving yourself? Every time he set a goal he reached it. Perfectly! Was I supposed to be upset by that? Doesn't every parent want her child to set goals and reach them successfully?
—Blanche Landow, age 46
Parent of recovering
anorexic son

Yes, all parents want their children to set and reach goals successfully. If a goal is realistic and healthy, then you can applaud you child's efforts to achieve. If your child is determined to win a race, get a part in a play, sing or play an instrument, excel academically, or be the best lawn-care specialist on the block, he or she may put an enormous amount of time, effort, and thought into achieving that goal. Intense and focused effort is healthy, unless the pursuit of the goal gets in the way of other goals or important relationships.

For example, one of your goals as a parent is to help your child understand how to maintain a healthy diet. You have this goal because you understand that eating properly helps you stay healthy and strong enough to grow and to build other aspects of your life. A good diet will help you be whatever you want, but it is not the kind of goal that should take up so much time, effort, and creativity that it interferes with a person's chance to achieve other goals and to enjoy life. So you have a goal to help your child learn to eat properly. But if you spend every hour of every day planning how to achieve that goal, it will eventually be more important than your child—or anything else.

You can see that the problem is not simply a matter of setting a goal. It's a matter of keeping the goal in perspective. If the goal becomes more important than the people you love, then there is a problem. If a goal like eating a particular food or reaching a specific weight stops you from achieving other things, then it's time to reevaluate why food and weight are more important to you than other projects, people, or life itself. You can see that if your goal to organize your food intake or lose weight becomes more important than your health, the whole point of dieting and exercising is defeated.

So the answer is "Yes, it's good for your children to learn how to set and achieve goals. And yes, it's okay for parents to express and act on that concern if the goal seems to be unhealthy." So trust yourself. If something about the way your child deals with food worries you, then you have nothing to lose by talking with your child, asking a doctor, checking with a specialist, or going to the library or bookstore to find reading material that will give you the information you need to be helpful for everyone concerned—including yourself.

Basically, it's hard to tell which is more difficult: growing up, or helping someone else grow up. When we think about how our own parents were and are, we may wonder why they fail to notice what we think or feel. And when we think about our children, we wonder how they can be so difficult to understand. Since we are simply human, we cannot expect our parents to understand us automatically or easily. By the same token, we cannot expect to understand our children's needs and feelings automatically.

As a family grows and changes, the needs and feelings of each person in that family change. But if you're accustomed to thinking of one another in just one way, then it's hard to see that the changes are taking place. Even if we see our children every day, it's difficult to see the changes or the problems that may be developing.

That's often because life gets so confusing and hectic. Your children may go from school to home, to play, or out to work. Or they may go to visit friends or take care of family business. You have to take care of your children's ordinary needs, and that means food, clothing, medical care, and all the comforts that go into making you and your child feel and look good. There is so much that has to be organized, maintained, and adjusted, it can be difficult to make time simply to be with each other.

With all the projects, activities, worries, and unanticipated problems that come up every day, it can be next to impossible for a parent to notice or understand symptoms of eating disorders, especially since those symptoms can develop little by little, day by day. And if you initially approved of the dieting or exercising, then you may find it difficult to withdraw your approval, especially if your child seems pleased with his or her accomplishments.

It could also be that you and your child have a hard time talking with each other about anything, much less about something sensitive and important. If that's the case, you may avoid saying anything directly to your youngster, even if you do notice that something may be wrong.

Then, if your child does develop a problem as grave as anorexia, bulimia, or bulimarexia, you may feel angry, guilty, confused, and overwhelmed. You wonder what you could or should have done differently, and you wonder how to help. You may call doctors or friends, read books, watch TV shows, or you may stay quiet about the whole thing, hoping that it will go away if you ignore it. But whether you choose to ignore or attack the problem, you probably have questions, like the ones Carl and Nancy Delacorte faced recently, about his 23-year-old daughter who lives in an apartment he and his wife built for her, at her request, in the basement of the home they have lived in all their lives.

Focusing on the Future: One Route to Recovery

My wife and I agreed on this—we both thought Jenny was bulimic. We saw the lists of all the different foods—and we knew she went out food shopping at odd hours. She came back with bags of food, but then she'd come up the next day because she didn't have anything left to eat. We didn't really know where to go with this thing at first. I mean, she wasn't a little kid anymore.... We didn't talk to her about it at first. We didn't know what to say. We didn't know if we should ask, because we didn't want her to think that we were prying. It was hard to tell what she was thinking, and we didn't know how she would feel if we said anything to her.

—Carl Delacorte, age 53
Father of recovering
bulimic daughter

It is perfectly normal to wonder how to parent a son or daughter who is over 18 or 21, and living at home. Parenting is confusing under the best of circumstances, and it can become overwhelming when you think an older child is suffering from a problem that could be dangerous.

At first, Carl and his wife, Nancy, responded to Jenny's problem by avoiding any kind of direct discussion about the issue, except between themselves. The fact was that Jenny knew that her parents could see when she went out, and when she went shopping. Sometimes her parents would greet her on her way in. So they all knew that she shopped very often, very heavily, and at strange hours. But no one said anything about it, because her parents were afraid of how Jenny would feel about their questions and concern, and Jenny was not ready to ask for help on her own.

Her shopping was not the only clue. There were the food lists—the good food/bad food behavior. Her parents never asked her about them, even though she hung them very openly on the refrigerator and the cabinets. Jenny was very rigid about what she would and would not eat in her parents' kitchen, but they decided to just ignore the behavior, because they did not know quite what to say. They only knew they were worried.

There's nothing simple about facing your child with that kind of concern. But every day, Carl and his wife were doing something much more difficult. They were carrying around the fear that they might find their daughter dead on the cold bathroom tile in her brand-new apartment. And they had other fears, as well. They thought that as long as Jenny lived with them, she was close to help she might need if she did get very sick. They were afraid she would move if they faced her on this issue—that she would move into a run-down apartment in a bad neighborhood because she could not afford decent rent. Then, if she did need them, it would take longer for them to reach her.

For months, they struggled with choices. Should they talk to her and risk seeing her move out in anger? Or should they keep avoiding the topic and stay close enough to help her in case something terrible happened to scare her into getting help.

They knew they were right when they argued it was impossible to anticipate what Jenny would do or say. But they also knew that they could not anticipate whether Jenny would live or die. And they lived with that conflict and fear every day.

The problems became more clear and unavoidable every day. There was more to Jenny's attitude and behavior than her shopping and her eating. There was the change in the way she was relating to people. She could be very abrupt, for no apparent reason. Her moods were intense and unpredictable, and she made her parents nervous. When Carl started to clean up their garbage after a dog knocked it over, he saw dozens of packets of water pills and laxatives in his daughter's trash. He was stunned. Jenny saw him cleaning up the trash and helped him, so she knew what he saw. But he never mentioned it, because he just did not know what to say. They simply complained to each other about the neighborhood dogs, and they both went their separate ways to work.

Carl talked with his wife, talked to a friend, called up a doctor, and started to gather information. He went to the local library and took out some books, and he called an eating disorders hotline to find a support group for parents of people with bulimia. After days of thinking and talking it over, Carl and his wife decided to go to that support group. Just listening to other people in similar circumstances gave them the courage and strength they needed to talk with their daughter, face to face.

I couldn't believe it. She denied everything. She even denied doing things she knew we knew about. That's when I knew she was in bad trouble. It was like she was saying that night was day. So we decided that we would confront her when she was really in trouble. We didn't spy on her or hang over her. We just let her be herself. And when she came in from a shopping trip, we waited about 20 minutes. Then we walked into her apartment without knocking.

You may think that was a violation of her privacy, but that thing she was doing was a violation of her body. You can't expect to survive an assault when you attack yourself with deadly force. And that's what she was doing. My God, she just dissolved. Right in the middle of the floor, surrounded by all these boxes and bags of junk food....She begged and pleaded for us to forgive her....I was staggered. I had prepared for the scene, but it was nothing like I expected. You just can't imagine. My beautiful daughter, on the floor at my feet, shaking and crying....

I lifted her to her feet, and we hugged her. We hugged her and told her we would always be there for her, but she needed to get help. They told us in the support group to let her know that we were there for her if she wanted to recover, but we would not stand by and watch her kill herself. We kept on telling her, "There's nothing to forgive. You're sick...you're not guilty of anything. You're just sick," but she kept on begging us to forgive her, and sobbing. We did everything the other parents talked about, and it worked. We told her that we knew, and we made her agree to go for help.

I wish I could tell you that everything went as smooth as silk, but it didn't. It was horrible. It was another two months and dozens of confrontations before she finally went to any doctor. And before she found the right kind of help for her, she went through so many changes. She got interested in a man who had a prison record and started to spend nights at his house. We were heartbroken, and I have to tell you we blamed each other. I blamed my wife for not letting me confront her earlier, and she blamed me for confronting her at all. I swear, sometimes I felt like I was losing my mind.

You know, my wife and I were always so close. We have always loved spending time with each other, and I'm proud of that relationship. You know, I never had another woman but her since I've been married? And we go everywhere together. She invites me to her social events, and I invite her to mine. We just love each other. And then this thing with my daughter started, and we fought terribly for the first time in our lives.

Now, I think maybe the group therapist was right. Maybe Jenny felt that we couldn't love her as much as we loved each other, and that would have made her angry. Maybe she thought we would abandon her—run away with each other, or just ignore her. I don't know. We have talked about that part of our lives, but I'm not sure yet how she felt. I'm actually not sure how she feels right now, but I'm less anxious, since she's really getting help. Back then, when she was getting involved with different men and rebelling worse than ever, I blamed myself, my wife, the neighborhood, my job, the schools, the teachers... everyone.... I was really out of control on this topic.

I want you to understand, I don't feel guilty anymore. I did in the beginning. In the beginning, I blamed everything we ever did. I kept trying to rethink camping trips and family trips—school nights I went to and school nights I missed. I mean, I drove myself out of my mind. I kept going over and over this kind of thing until I thought I would go crazy. Then one night in the group therapy for parents, this one father kept saying how he felt responsible for the whole problem, and his wife agreed.

Suddenly, I saw red. I shouted out, "You are not responsible! Maybe you did things inadvertently that hurt your son, but you damn sure didn't mean to make him sick. Now you're trying to change, so stop torturing yourself. He's got to take some responsibility for getting better, too. You can't do it for him!"

As soon as all that came out of me, I realized I was really talking about myself and my wife. And I was talking about my daughter, not that man's son. That's when I knew we could all really be okay. That support group was a lifesaver for us....

When we look at Jenny today, it's hard to believe that we went through all that. She's back in her apartment, paying us rent and utilities, and she's going to the doctor every week. The change is incredible. Sure, she's had slips. And would you believe it? She admits them. When she gets really nervous and she forgets to do the relaxation exercises, sometimes she slips back. But she's able to stop after one episode, and the time between episodes is months, not hours.

Today, I believe that my daughter will get well. She's got certain problems with her bodily functions because of the way she abused herself, but medical doctors are working with her on that. And these days, when she feels good or excited or bad or worried, she talks with someone. Sometimes it's us, sometimes it isn't. But she doesn't need to stuff her feelings down her throat and then try to flush them out of her body and down the toilet, or wash them away in the shower. You can't destroy or ignore feelings like self-hatred or powerlessness, because they just get worse. Feelings are a part of you, so you may as well get in touch with them.... I can tell you one thing... These days, I'm feeling pretty damn good, and I've been telling everyone.

Carl feels ''pretty damn good'' because he decided to find out whether he could do something to help himself, his wife, and his daughter. He's proud that his family could face such a crisis and come out better and stronger than ever.

Basically, Carl and his wife went through some very specific steps to help their daughter and themselves.

Twelve Steps Toward Recovery

1. They admitted that their daughter had an eating disorder.

2. They admitted that the eating disorder was too powerful for them or their daughter to cope with alone.

3. They gathered information about eating disorders.

4. They made lists of doctors and organizations specializing in helping individuals and families understand and defeat eating disorders.

5. They shared their concern with their daughter.

6. They persisted in sharing that concern, even when their daughter vigorously denied that she was bulimic.

7. They got help for themselves through a support group.

8. They relied on each other and on the support group to help them stand firm when their daughter seemed to get worse before she got better.

9. They were willing to change the way they dealt with stress in the family.

10. They were willing to give up guilt and blame and to start experimenting with new ways of relating to each other.

11. They accepted the fact that their whole family would change if their daughter changed.

12. They learned that change doesn't just happen: It can evolve slowly, a little bit at a time, and each little bit is cause for celebration, because the big changes are made up of all the small failures and successes that are part of healing.

When the Delacortes admitted that their daughter had an eating disorder, they could concentrate on that one problem without getting distracted by other medical or social problems that their daughter may have suffered because of the eating disorder. It was crucial for them to admit that the eating disorder was stronger than either themselves or their daughter, because that prepared them to accept information and help. They were not used to asking for help, and that particular step toward understanding and defeating bulimia was crucial.

The information they gathered about eating disorders made them feel more confident when they took the fifth step and faced their daughter. They did not want to approach her from a position of ignorance, because they knew that she had read volumes of books on nutrition and diet. Without their own resources and information, they would have felt helpless when their daughter denied having any problems with food or feelings.

The information they got helped them persist in sharing that concern, and the professional help they sought gave them the encouragement they needed to remain persistent. They also learned that if their daughter started to change, they would change, too. It's a natural process. If one member of a group begins to act differently yet remains with the group, then the other members tend to act differently, too—and a family is a group. So they were willing to direct energy and effort to changing in a positive direction.

Because they understood the nature of the disorder, Carl and Nancy were able to give up all the guilt and blame that had interfered with their relationship and made life at home tense and unhappy. Once they gave up guilt and blame, they were free to concentrate on learning new ways to talk and be with each other. That willingness to find new ways to relate to one another has become the foundation for the future of that family. It can become the foundation for yours, as well, if you accept that recovery is a process that takes time, energy, and faith.

13 | How Every Teacher Can Help

Roberta Richin, M.A.

I went into teaching because I really enjoyed the work. I wanted to teach kids, but to tell you the truth, I don't know what I'm expected to do these days. I have at least 25 kids in every class, and I teach five classes a day. I have to do lesson plans, correct and review homework, correct and review tests, do mountains of paper work, meet with parents, go to school myself....I have 125 kids, and I'm supposed to see which ones are abused or suicidal, self-destructive, into drugs or alcohol—and now you want me to know about kids with eating disorders. I'm a teacher. I have to do the job I was hired to do: teach. How can I teach, and help all these kids you say are in some sort of trouble?

—Al Presser
Social Studies teacher,
Grades 10 and 11

Walk into a faculty room or education course, and you will probably find people debating how, when, why, and to what extent teachers should respond to or inquire into various aspects of a child's private life. For example, legislation has mandated that all teachers and other school professionals respond to the problem of child abuse and maltreatment by reporting their suspicions to government agencies. Other legislation and social programs variously urge teachers to help children who may appear depressed, anxious, self-destructive, suicidal, drug involved, learning disabled, emotionally disturbed, or otherwise at risk of becoming adults who are not successful, contributing members of the society. At the same time, legislative and professional initiatives continue to legitimately emphasize that teachers are responsible for producing competent students year after year, under conditions where student achievement can be measured by standardized tests.

Therefore, schools appear to be operating under two mandates: (1) To concentrate on instructional gains, so the students acquire specific knowledge that can be measured by testing; and (2) to concentrate on helping students overcome emotional, behavioral, psychological, or medical difficulties that may interfere with the student's ability to learn and grow.

With these two distinct but interdependent mandates, teaching has become a profession in transition. Teachers, like doctors, are increasingly required to make unprecedented choices based on legal requirements, available technology, and moral imperatives. Just as doctors can be trained to balance those various and compelling interests, so can teachers. With appropriate education and support, teachers can and often already do teach their students traditional subject matter while satisfying the social and legal expectations that require teachers to protect and nurture children so they can succeed in school and in the community.

To accomplish such a complex task, teachers need an updated job description. That job description must be based on a clear definition of the teacher's role as it relates to the child, the child's family, and the community. It is not sufficient simply to train a teacher how to identify children who present such pressing and dangerous problems as eating disorders or other life-threatening conditions. That teacher must clearly understand how to act on that knowledge so that the integrity and safety of each teacher, family, school, community, and child are protected.

Figuring Out Where You Fit In: One Point of View

If you're a teacher, it's hard to figure out where you fit in. You know you're supposed to be in the classroom, teaching the subjects and skills you were trained to impart. But then there are the special problems. Like the 14-year-old boy who seems to be bulimic because he wants to eat like the other guys and still be in the right weight class on the wrestling team. Or the 16-year-old straight-A student who tells you she is pregnant and her father is the father of her baby.

You may find out that your fourth-grade student who is just borderline between passing and failing has been coming in late because he has to get his younger sister ready for school on the days when their mom and dad are drunk. And even though you may never have heard of anorexia, you may feel more and more worried about your super student who looks as if she is simply starving to death.

When you look around your classroom at youngsters in need of services beyond the scope of your training, you may wonder "Is this my business? Or is this family business?" The answer is clear: *It's your business because it's more than family business. Here is the framework for your rationale:*

The relationship between parent and child is not absolute. It is defined by social norms, religious convictions, and legal mandates. Children are no longer considered the property of their parents. Rather, they are in trust to their parents. Society charges parents with the responsibility of caring for children so that the children will eventually become capable of taking care of themselves and contributing positively to the larger society.

That may seem simple and obvious enough, but there is really nothing simple or obvious about parenting. It's a huge task that virtually everyone has trouble with at one time or another. Every family experiences a wide range of success and defeat, and every family has problems. Sometimes it's relatively easy for a family to identify the fact that there is a problem and to then gather the information, skills, and support necessary to solve the problem.

For example, if a youngster suddenly starts to limp or complain that his leg hurts, his mother or father would probably have his leg examined by a doctor. If that mother or father did not have enough experience, knowledge, or resources to understand that the child's leg could be fixed, then the child would not get medical attention. The quality of that child's life might be permanently damaged, unless a teacher or other concerned professional in a position of authority could help the parents see that there was a problem, and that it could be solved.

In that scenario, the teacher would not presume to actually fix the child's leg. He or she would simply act as an informed link between the family and the appropriate support service available. That child would have a healthy leg, and a better life, because the teacher shared her information with the child's parents and helped the parents understand how and where to get help for their child, and perhaps for the rest of the family.

The analogy fits any and every other situation where a child's health or welfare lies in the balance. Teachers who are trained to identify children who might need attention from medical doctors, psychotherapists, or other professionals serve the children, the school, the family, and the community by acting as an informed link between the family and the resource that can help.

When a teacher is trained to identify a child in need, the child is served because additional help is offered. In most instances, children and teenagers do not have the legal authority to seek help for themselves. They do not have the experience, skills, power, emotional capacity, social status, or knowledge always to seek the help they need. Because of their age and dependent status, they need their parents, teachers, religious leaders, and other important adults to help them get the assistance they require, so they can succeed in school and grow into self-sufficient adults in their own right.

When teachers are trained to identify children in need of help beyond the scope of traditional classroom or guidance services, the school is served in several ways. First, the school is protected from accusations that it failed to act on behalf of a child. Consider what might happen if a bulimic youngster experienced cardiac arrythmia and died in the locker room of a public school. The principal, coaches, classroom teachers, and counselors would probably be asked how a child could have engaged in such behavior without the knowledge or understanding of the school authorities. The child's life could have been saved if the teachers and other professionals involved with that child were trained to identify the problem and connect the youngster and perhaps the family to the help they would need.

When teachers serve as informed links between the youngster, the family, and appropriate services inside or outside the school, these teachers serve the school in a solidly traditional way: They help the child develop academically and socially. If a teacher links a youngster to an appropriate educational, medical or mental health service, then the child can have a chance to learn solid problem-solving skills and recover from a problem or illness. Many teachers report that youngsters who receive appropriate medical and psychological services enjoy academic and social success, often beyond their expected limits. On the other hand, children whose medical or psychological needs are neglected can suffer years of underachievement and behavior problems.

Children who suffer academic and behavior problems absorb an enormous amount of the teacher's time, energy, and resourcefulness. If a teacher is not prepared to identify a child in need and link the child and perhaps the family to suitable professional services, the teacher often ends up struggling unsuccessfully to control or motivate a child whose neglected problems become more entrenched every day. When that child underachieves or behaves inappropriately, he or she often distracts the class and the teacher.

George Atkins recalls the young man whose grades and behavior took a sudden turn for the worse in eleventh grade.

Jerry wasn't the best kid in the class, but he wasn't the worst. I teach math, and I'm used to kids struggling with the subject. So many of their parents were afraid of math, it's a miracle that the kids come in as optimistic and positive as they do. Jerry was right in the middle, a strong B or high C student when he did his homework, came to class, and concentrated on the lesson.

He was really a good kid: Participated in sports, came to class on time...put in an effort at everything he did. At the time, he was on the football team, and he wanted to play a particular position. I don't remember what it was, but he had to be heavier. So over the summer, during football training, he gained weight. I mean, he put on 20 pounds so fast it was incredible. When he came back to school, he looked really different. Some of it was muscle from working out, and some of it was fat.

Then, of course, he had to stop stuffing himself, because he reached the weight he wanted. I had never really paid attention to the whole weight and food dynamic, but he started to come late to my class. The class met just after lunch. Later, after this whole eating problem was revealed, I understood that he continued to stuff himself, but then he would go into the boys' locker room and throw up after he ate every bit of food he could get his hands on. But at the time, I was really concerned with the lateness, because lateness distracts the kid and the whole class, and it can lead to cutting.

So I warned him about the latenesses, but it didn't matter. The kids started expecting him to be late and laughing when he came in all flushed and short of breath. It became a real pattern with him, so I gave him detention. Those are the rules! I thought his eyes were watery and he was flushed and breathing hard because he was high. I thought he ate tons of junk food all the time because he was high on marijuana, and marijuana makes you want to eat that way. So I talked to the coach, who talked to him, and the coach got so frustrated because Jerry refused to say anything that the kid ended up getting suspended from the team. That finished it. He started to cut my class, and when he did come, he was disruptive and sarcastic....

I really should have referred him to the nurse the minute I thought anything was wrong. Now I know that I just don't have the training to diagnose everything, and it's impossible to tell what's wrong when a kid is acting even more strangely than usual. As soon as I have any reason to think a kid is high on marijuana, I refer him right to the nurse. How am I supposed to know what's wrong? Even if he did get high, how do I know what was really in the drug? It's all illegal or illegally acquired, anyway, so they have no idea what they're taking. And I sure don't know. So if a kid seems like he's high or feeling odd, he goes straight to the nurse. That way, he gets help, I can concentrate on teaching, and I have prevented an additional crisis or tragedy that could develop in the classroom if the kid suddenly falls down, faints, or loses control.

Anyway, I really didn't know where to go with the situation. I talked with his parents a few times on the telephone, and they were just as confused as I was. We figured he was going through a rebellious phase, so...since his schoolwork was suffering, his parents grounded him, and let him know—he had to shape up.

After he went from a B to an F in my class and failed the midterm, we had a parent/teacher conference. I dreaded that meeting, because I really didn't know what was going wrong. I felt he was drug involved, but I didn't want to tell that to the parents. So I described all of Jerry's different behaviors—

positive and negative—and they came to the same conclusion. They decided Jerry should go for counseling.

Meanwhile, the football season was long over, and Jerry went out for wrestling. Our school doesn't have eligibility requirements based on grades, so Jerry got on the team without a problem. His coach told him if he weighed just a little bit less, he could wrestle at the top of one weight class, instead of at the bottom of another one. If he could get some weight off and learned the right moves, he could be a real winner.

Well, he got that weight off 1—2—3. I remember saying that if he could lose weight like that, he should be able to do math, but it didn't sink in. One goal had nothing to do with the other. He was still failing math, and he started to fail English, his first-period class, because he was coming in late and disorganized—unprepared, distracted. He looked like he was high on something.

The therapist who was seeing Jerry gave me a call at school. She said that his parents had signed a release allowing her to talk with Jerry's teachers, and anything I had to say would be helpful. I was amazed that she called—mostly, I don't ever hear anything from psychologists or social workers. Anyway, it was just before I had to get to class, so I only talked a couple of minutes. Basically, I complained about the kid. I complained to her that if he set academic goals the way he set sports goals for himself, he'd be on the honor roll. She asked what I meant, and I said that he gains and loses weight so fast he could probably make a million dollars if he wrote down his diet, and he really puts in the effort for his coaches. Then I had to go to class. She thanked me and said I could call her anytime, and that she would be in touch.

I didn't think about it again for another week. We had third-quarter tests and grades to get done, and I've always found grading tough. It's hard to sum up a kid in one letter or one number. And it means so much to the kid. Anyway, in the middle of all this, on a Friday afternoon when I was on my way out of school to go get my son, who came home from college for the weekend, the school social worker stopped me in the main office. He said that Jerry's therapist had tried to reach me, but I was in class. Then he told me Jerry was bulimic.

I remember feeling so stupid. I didn't know what he meant. So I asked. I hadn't been all wrong. He was getting high on marijuana, but not between classes. The red eyes and flushed cheeks—and the junk food wrappers that were always stuffed in his pockets—those were all symptoms of the bulimia. He was late to first period and my class because that's when he would purge. He would go into the locker room bathroom when it cleared out and everyone was in the gym or on the field. That's why he was late. No one ever knew anything.

Of course, everything fell into place then. Hindsight is 20/20, right? He's been seeing this therapist for a few months now, and his grades are going up. He's also been coming to class on time. His weight hasn't changed, but that's probably a good sign. I'm not sure.

I'm only sure of one thing. Next time I have a kid who goes through some dramatic behavior changes, I'm going to write all those changes down, tell his parents right away, and refer him for counseling in the school or outside the school. I can't know everything that can happen to a kid, but I can make a record of what I see, and then I can refer the kid to someone who does know what I don't.

Just to let you know, Jerry did pass the class. He got a B in the fourth quarter, a C on the final exam, and a C for a final grade. Since he was a B/C student in general, it was cause for celebration. I was impressed that the kid could go through so much change and still pull it together in school. I think he still has some problems, but who doesn't? At least now, everyone's doing something, including him. And I have a successful student, instead of the disruptive, obnoxious kid he had become in the middle of the year.

* * *

Although George did not know the origin of Jerry's behavior and was not equipped to make any diagnosis, he refused to allow Jerry to fail or withdraw. George rejected the possibility that his student was involved in a vicious cycle of failure and poor behavior that he could not change. Basically, he acted on the assumptions that:

1. Jerry could achieve academic success in math.

2. Jerry could learn new coping skills to overcome his personal difficulties, which were found to include a serious eating disorder.

3. Jerry's parents could be included in the problem-identification process, because they are partners in Jerry's education.

4. Jerry's other teachers, coaches, counselors, and other school professionals could serve as resources to help Jerry reestablish himself as a functioning student.

5. Teachers can apply the same basic communications skills with emotionally needy children that they already apply when youngsters require medical care for injury or illness.

On the basis of these primary assumptions, George succeeded in his efforts to include the student, the parents, and other school professionals in his effort to help this particular student become more successful academically and behaviorally. The focus on academic and behavioral adjustment helped the family understand that many students go through personal crises that initially appear mysterious, but that can be understood and addressed when teachers, parents, and students develop a clear plan for action to initiate change.

According to George, Jerry's parents had a reputation for being defensive and difficult to reach. Despite that reputation, there was no choice: Jerry's academic and behavioral difficulties in math were such that parent/teacher contact would be inevitable. Given that such a meeting would have to take place, George carefully framed his initial statement to Jerry's parents, saying basically, "I know you share my interest in Jerry's success. I'm concerned about some changes that I see in Jerry, and I would like to let you know what they are. Perhaps you will understand them better than I do."

In that one brief opening statement to Jerry's parents, George accomplished three critical goals:

1. He offered the parents no choice but to agree that they are interested in their child's success.

2. He established a nonjudgmental tone of concern.

3. He resisted the impulse to ask whether there were problems at home and focused instead on suggesting his willingness to rely on the parents for insight and partnership in problem solving.

At no point did George attempt to diagnose the problem for the parents or the student. He did not accuse the boy of drug involvement, and he did not call the parents with a message that they had failed in some way. He simply acted on the belief that most students placed in his class belonged in his class and could learn the material. George also understood that even the most confusing and irritating behavioral problems are generally an indication that the student is having some sort of difficulty that might be too personal or complex for a classroom teacher to either diagnose or treat.

The core of George's approach is simple: Teachers are professional people, trained to do a specific job. They are not trained to counsel individual students, and they are not trained to do family therapy. First and foremost, teachers are charged with the responsibility of empowering students to acquire and apply skills and knowledge.

As a teacher, you know you are not trained to diagnose emotional or psychological problems and should not be held responsible for treatment or diagnosis. You are, however, trained to record and report specific incidents, behavior changes, academic developments, and learning problems. And you do need communication skills that will help you listen to, process, and respond to problems that you observe, or that other people report to you.

George was put in a position that you will recognize immediately if you are a teacher: He had to try to teach a youngster who was resistant and angry. If George had tried to counsel Jerry, where would he have started? How would he have tested the accuracy of his diagnosis? When would he have involved the parents, and how would he have explained that he tried to counsel the boy despite the fact that his training is limited to math and science education?

Think About What Would Happen If a Youngster Got Injured Under Your Supervision

If a student falls down and breaks a bone, you know precisely what to do. You make absolutely sure that the youngster receives prompt, professional medical attention, usually through the school nurse. Depending on your school policy, the nurse, classroom teacher, or administrator notifies the parent while emergency medical care is provided. Unless you are a medical doctor, Emergency Medical Technician, or other trained medical services professional, you would never even attempt to manipulate or set the bone, because you know that you could cause serious and even permanent damage. But that does not mean you're helpless. You would make informed, timely decisions to get the youngster the right care. Then you would try to make the child feel safe and comfortable while he or she is waiting for professional help.

Never would you tell an injured child to sit in the back of the class with his face to the wall so you could finish your lesson. And you would not lecture him that it was all his own fault, so he should stand on his own two feet and take care of the problem by himself, since you are a teacher and not trained to help. You would automatically be supportive, say you understand that he is pain, and assure him that he will be okay so long as he allows trained professionals to help him and eventually helps himself.

When that injured or sick youngster comes back to class, his condition may dictate that you modify some expectations and keep other expectations high. Perhaps you would talk with the student, his parents, and even his doctor, so you could determine just how high those expectations should be at each phase of recovery. You know that it would help him tackle the challenge of school if you acknowledge that his situation or problem might be uncomfortable or stressful, but that you are confident he can keep on learning at an appropriate pace, in spite of physical discomfort, frustration with the problem, or some other related difficulty. You would expect the youngster to tell you if he was tired, overwhelmed, or needed more of a challenge. And you would pay attention to those messages, so he could continue to achieve and grow.

No matter what grade or subject you teach, you have probably had a student who required some professional help to recover from an injury or physical illness. There is virtually no difference between the way you would respond to obvious medical emergencies or physical problems, and the way you would react when children present other kinds of special needs that require professional help that you have not been trained to administer.

If you stay informed about the child's progress and needs, and you let that youngster know that you believe he can continue to learn and develop, then you are part of the solution. You are helping the child recover precisely because you are staying on task—empowering your student to get needed help, overcome difficulties, problem solve, and achieve. By accomplishing those goals, you fulfill your contract with the school and community, and you stay within the confines of your professional training.

Fitting Into a Service Network

As a classroom teacher, George Atkins feels confident that he did what he could to identify a potential problem, refer a youngster for help, and then get back on task. His actions were designed to help him protect the student, cover himself, concentrate on instruction, and supply the parents with sufficient nonjudgmental information so they could ensure that their son would receive the appropriate care and support.

In that fashion, George served as an informed link between parent and child. Since then, he has gathered information about local youth and family services and treatment for young people who suffer from eating disorders and other life-threatening problems. With that information, George can now approach parents, students, and colleagues with more confidence, because he knows more about resources and how to refer people to those resources. He does not confuse referral with treatment, and he feels more powerful, because he is better informed. Now he can serve as an informed link between young people in need, their families, and the appropriate private, public, or school services.

In the midst of all the pressure on classroom teachers to be so many things to so many students, George Atkins has finally been able to determine where he fits. He feels comfortable in the classroom again, because he is teaching youngsters math and referring them for help in those cases where the student requires help George is not trained to provide. Today, he sees himself as part of a whole network of professionals who can help youngsters. He no longer feels that he's solely responsible for making sure the student achieves according to expected learning ability. As part of a network of professionals serving the instructional, developmental, social, and health needs of children and families, he feels much more confident and content in his role as a teacher.

Once You Know Where You Fit: A Practical Guide for Action

If you are a teacher, you have attended seminars and training courses designed to help you understand and identify children at risk of special problems, including self-destructive behavior, drug involvement, abuse or maltreatment, and eating disorders, to name only a few. As an informed link between parents, students, and in-school or out-of-school treatment or prevention programs, it would be appropriate for you to help connect parents and youngsters to suitable agencies or individuals. But how do you accomplish that task, and still get everything else done? How do you act as an informed link and avoid incurring the wrath of parents, your supervisor, principals, or school board members?

Although life is full of twists and turns that make it important to adjust plans of action from time to time, there are certain steps you can take to protect yourself, the youngster in need, and the integrity of the instructional process.

1. Keep a specific, detailed record of the student's behavior or record of achievement, so you are always prepared to present a coherent report if you or someone else initiates a parent/teacher conference.

2. Alert your supervisor to your concerns and to any action you may take to talk with parents or refer the student for other help.

3. Address any supervisor's concern about your role as a referral source by (a) referring the parent to more than one individual or agency and (b) discussing with that supervisor what might happen to the child and the school if the referral or parent contact is not made—for example, student illness on school grounds, progression of student's problems into other areas, making the child a danger to himself or others at school.

4. Understand that the child is an extension of the parents, and the parents are likely to be either defensive, embarrassed, intensely worried, or so distracted by other difficulties that they may appear to be unconcerned. Therefore, expect only that information will help the parents function more effectively, and do not judge parental love or interest on the basis of just a few parent/teacher contacts.

5. Understand that parents often experience anxiety when they go to parent/teacher conferences. You can treat parents as guests in your professional environment when you:

- Meet them at the front door of the school.
- Show them where their child sits in your class.
- Sit on the same side of the desk as they are sitting, except if they are threatening to you.
- Set a time limit for the meeting and share that limit with the parents.
- Agree on an agenda for the meeting.
- Discuss, not lecture about, your special concern about their child.
- Share information you have gathered about their child.
- Ask the parents for input rather than telling the parents what you think they should do for the student.
- Agree on specific shared goals for the youngster.
- Make sure the parents understand the goals by having them help you clarify just what you have all agreed to accomplish.
- If you agree on a plan, write it down to determine good evaluation points—for example, one week to contact the doctor and then a follow-up parent/teacher contact for mutual support and insight.
- If you do not agree on a plan, schedule a second meeting to include the school social worker, principal, and other relevant professionals to pursue the issue from a different direction.
- Terminate the meeting on time, with a plan for future contact.
- Notify your supervisor of the progress that was or was not made in the meeting.

* * *

If you apply that basic process for parent/teacher contact regarding concerns as grave as eating disorders, you can be confident that you will inform yourself, inform the parents, protect yourself, protect your supervisor, protect the student, and concentrate on teaching.

When David Meyer, a music teacher for elementary school children, was told that one of his former orchestra students had been hospitalized for anorexia, he recalled how he used to worry about her.

She used to put extra hours and hours into rehearsal, demanding more of herself than anyone else expected. One of my colleagues from the high school stopped by while she was practicing a solo, and he said he wished he had a whole class like that. I didn't. I thought there was something wrong. It's okay to pursue perfection if you know you're human, and you know you'll only achieve it to a degree. With Candy, there was no such thing as success. There was only the next goal.

We do all the normal things here... Christmas concerts and Spring shows... She played flute, and she was very good. Technically, that is. There was another child in orchestra who played like she was born to the instrument. It was incredible. The other kids used to sit and listen to her with real respect and admiration. Hey, so did I. I could never be as good. That kid has a real future. Candy was good, but she wasn't marvelous in the same way. You know how I told you that the other kids would listen and admire the child? Well, Candy would cry. Hysterically. I mean, she would sob, all by herself, in a corner, once she thought everyone was gone. I found her like that twice, and both times she apologized profusely, as if she had committed a crime... said it wouldn't happen again. I told her she had nothing to apologize for, and I asked if there was anything I could do. She said, "No. I have to do it. I just have to."

I figured it was just a phase. And you have to understand, I teach all the children in this school. That means I have 741 children, grades kindergarten through sixth grade. I see them once a week, for 43 minutes, and then I see others for orchestra or other lessons. If I jumped every time a sixth-grade girl cried, I would be like a Mexican jumping bean.

On the other hand, I have to admit...I felt there was something wrong. I talked to a couple of other teachers, and I even talked to the school psychologist. It went as far as them looking up her records to see what her other teachers had observed about her, and they all said the same thing: "A perfect pleasure!" A perfect pleasure. We were so right. It was impossible for anyone to put out that energy to please so many of us so completely, and still grow up. Growing up means that you're a pain in the neck to someone at some point. But this kid made everyone happy.

I wish I knew then what I know now. I would have pursued it...talked with her parents...let them know I was worried about how pressured the kid was. They were really good people, and they respected us. I think that I could have made them at least feel the same worry I was feeling, enough so they would explore the problem with a doctor. After all, they were her parents.

You are in a position to effectively save your students, their families, yourself, and your other students from the desperate and dangerous situation faced by David Meyer, Candy, and Candy's family. You can concentrate on reaching your instructional goals and still equip yourself, your students, their parents, and your supervisors with the information and insight that can literally save lives.

Try the referral process. Hang topical support service posters featuring hotline telephone numbers on your bulletin boards. And know that many of the students you struggle to serve and empower are carrying burdens so heavy that they can become literally immobilized. Although you may not know how to help that student with the particular problem, you can connect that boy or girl and even the family to the resource that can help so that you and your student can get back to the business of teaching and learning.

Answers to Questions That Always Come Up

How do I make a referral if my school policy says that I cannot make such a move without a counselor or supervisor being part of the process?

If your school district or building policy restrains you from making a referral based on a thorough understanding of local community resources, then you may feel that you are caught between a rock and a hard place. In many ways, you are the one who is responsible for the student. You are held accountable if the student fails or achieves, and you are generally held accountable for answers and information in those tense encounters between parents, principals, counselors, and you, when the student in question is already in considerable academic, social, or emotional difficulty.

You know the scenario. A reasonably competent student with a solid record of achievement is presenting behavior or academic problems that are simply uncharacteristic. Maybe the changes took place slowly, and you did not notice at first. Or the changes may have developed very rapidly, and you were so surprised that you decided to see if the problem would go away as quickly as it developed.

If positive change does not develop spontaneously as youngsters go through various developmental stages, you may begin to extend yourself to that student. Maybe you offer extra help, or a sympathetic ear. You may try to reason with the boy or girl if the problem involves cutting classes, inappropriate behavior, or achievement that falls significantly below the student's ability.

As soon as the student presents the difficulty, you begin to react, and the dynamic between you, the youngster, and perhaps the rest of the class causes you stress. So you may spend five weeks or eight weeks trying to cope with the student yourself. If your efforts are unsuccessful, you may then attempt to contact the parents. At that point, your stress and anxiety level regarding the youngster's classroom problems is much higher than that of the parents, because you have been carrying the burden of solving the problem all by yourself.

By the same token, if you spend five or eight weeks attempting to resolve the issues on your own, and then go to your department chairperson, dean, assistant principal, guidance counselor, or principal, your feelings are much more intense than his or hers will be at first. After all, this is the first time that person is hearing something specific from you about this particular student. He or she cannot be expected to feel as intensely as you do about the issue, because he or she has not received the same exposure to the difficulty that you have received, day in and day out, in each and every class the student has attended.

If your school policy dictates that you cannot make a referral on your own, then you have to first identify the person who is your designated partner in providing the support service to that youngster. Is it the assistant principal? The school social worker? The building principal? Your department chairperson?

That designated partner varies from district to district and building to building. If you do not know who it is, find out. If you do not like or respect the person, try to identify an alternative partner. If you do not have a choice, then you must come to terms with the fact that you are likely to have to work side by side with that person at some point or other. It may as well be in a situation where you are prepared, and where you initiate the action.

Whether or not you like or respect the person you must work with, you still have to follow procedure. If you fail to follow procedure, you make yourself vulnerable. If you are vulnerable, you cannot serve the student effectively. Therefore, following procedure keeps you and your student out of jeopardy.

Once you know who your partner in problem solving may be, you share your perspective on the child from the very beginning of the process. You jot down a memo, or fill out an appropriate form, notifying the person that the student is presenting a specific behavior or attitude, and you are addressing it in a specific way. Document your actions. Do not simply lean into an office, or talk briefly over lunch or coffee, and expect that person to remember what you said, when you said it, or why.

First, you would make an appointment to see your supervisor. The appointment can last just five or ten minutes, but it is formal, there is a record of it, and it calls special attention to the fact that you are appropriately sharing what you are doing to help the student. You are also seeking supervision in the process. In this fashion you immediately begin to share responsibility for the student with the partner that your school says shares responsibility. You are also making sure that your partner is being exposed to the entire process, including your efforts and the student's struggle to cooperate with you or to resist you.

This process cuts through your very real isolation in that classroom and gives you the support and documentation you may need when it comes time to defend what you have done to help a child. If your supervisor is privy to what you have done, knows how and when you contacted parents and why you initiated certain actions, then you and the student are protected. If you decide on your own to initiate action, appeal to the student in an unorthodox way, break or bend rules for the youngster, or reach out to the parents without documenting what you said and when you said it, then you may find yourself in the unenviable position of defending your actions to a supervisor who did not know what you were doing.

A principal in a Long Island, New York, school district urges all teachers to understand that a supervisor who knows and approves of what you are doing to help a student overcome a difficulty is a supervisor you can count on to support you when and if it becomes necessary for you to explain your actions to parents or other concerned parties.

If I have a student who is going through some sort of psychological or medical therapy, what is my role in helping the youngster succeed in school?

Privacy is a critical issue for any person receiving medical or psychological services. Very often, parents, counselors, psychologists, medical doctors, social workers, principals, and even the students themselves will feel that the teacher should not necessarily know the nature of the youngster's difficulty. The matter really should be decided on an individual basis. Teachers who are told about a student's particular problem must also get some direction regarding, first, what kind of behavior the student may present, and second, how best to respond to that behavior in order to support the therapeutic goals while still supporting the instructional and educational goals of the school.

If a student is anorexic, for example, it would be helpful for all the teachers, including the physical education teacher, to know that:

● The youngster has an eating disorder that could kill her.
● Perfectionism is a big part of the problem.
● Teachers should not continually reinforce that particular student's efforts to lose weight, get absolutely perfect scores, or run errands and do chores that will ingratiate her to adults.
● People who develop eating disorders can interpret even casual remarks about their weight as permission to begin and maintain a life-threatening attitude toward food, fat, and exercise.

Basically, teachers can reinforce and support therapeutic goals if they are privy to those goals.

Three basic steps can and should be taken in situations where teachers can reinforce therapeutic goals:

● First, the parent must sign a release for the therapist stating that the therapist may discuss specific aspects of the youngster's needs with the teachers or other school professionals. The parent and therapist can agree ahead of time on exactly what to disclose and whom to disclose it to, based on their understanding of what a teacher can respond to in the context of the classroom.

● Second, the therapist must understand that the teacher's primary goal and responsibility is to help the student master the skills or subject being taught.

● Third, the therapist, teacher, parent, and youngster can agree on a procedure that allows the classroom teacher to:

    1. Target short-term goals to improve in specific problem areas that may exist in class.

    2. Establish a time-frame within which the goals will be evaluated.

    3. Establish criteria for evaluating how much of the goal has been achieved.

    4. Understand that all achievement involves process, and that incremental achievement must be recognized and rewarded.

Whenever teachers, parents, students, counselors, principals, or psychotherapists develop a plan to help a youngster improve some aspect of school adjustment or achievement, it is crucial for everyone involved to understand that change is a process, just like a journey. If you build a plan based on the expectation that a student will change directly from being completely distracted in class to being completely focused on the material being presented, then everyone will be disappointed, because the student will fail. The goal is simply too big.

However, if you build a plan based on the clear understanding that the student can increase the amount of time spent on-task, attentive, and relaxed, then you and everyone involved can experience success, because the key word is "increase." It may help if you think about a youngster's improvement program as a journey. If you set out to drive from New York to California, you know that it will take you time to reach your goal. You know you may get lost along the way. You know there may be some unexpected developments, like road work or errors in directions, and you also know that you can count on markers, like road signs, that will let you know you are making progress along the right road.

You may choose a route that will take you from New York, through New Jersey and Pennsylvania, and into Ohio. You would expect to progress at a certain rate toward your goal, and you would never expect to get to California without going through the states between your origin and your destination, one by one. You would not start punishing yourself and feeling bad because you had been driving for nine hours and had only reached Ohio. You would not feel disappointed that you were driving for a day and had not yet reached your goal.

And even after you did get to California, you would understand that it is a very large state, with thousands of streets and sights and perspectives to know and enjoy. You would not expect to get to a new state and immediately feel as comfortable as if you were in the place that used to be so familiar. So the whole process takes time.

Changing from one personal or school-based behavior or attitude to another is the same as moving from one state to another. It involves information, planning, time, support, and a built-in way to evaluate progress over time. If we all embraced positive change without resistance, then we would not have difficulty with diets, exercise programs, smoking, seatbelts, disorganization, personal relationships, or change in the workplace. We would simply adopt any and all behaviors that we knew would make us happier, healthier, wealthier, or more productive.

The reality is that we find change scary, even when it's good.

Change causes us anxiety as adults, and it causes us anxiety as youngsters, too. When we ask students to change their behavior, attitudes, or skills in order to be more successful and complete people, they will probably experience a variety of feelings about change. The range of feelings would be a key topic to discuss with a student's psychotherapist, in order to better understand how a youngster may feel happy, anxious, hopeful, doubtful, and frightened all at the same time, in reaction to the idea that he or she can change and improve.

Youngsters receiving treatment for an eating disorder may be virtually terrified at the notion of change. With the permission of the parent, the psychotherapist may work with you to develop strategies that can target and support both therapeutic and instructional goals for such a student. It is ultimately up to the child's parents to determine how much of that student's background is disclosed to you. Very often it is simply unnecessary for you to know certain aspects of a student's background. After all, you are a professional in your own right. You have to set and achieve instructional and developmental goals for the students in your care, and you cannot be expected to absorb and react to personal information about all the students you have who may be in therapy.

If the child's therapist or medical doctor contacts you, then you can expect that the parents have agreed to let you understand certain aspects of the child's background and current status. You can also expect to work together with that health professional to set, evaluate, and possibly revise goals and objectives for that youngster in your classroom. You may find the doctor a valuable resource in helping you develop different ways of dealing with behavior that you find irritating, perplexing, or unmanageable.

If, on the other hand, the child's therapist or medical doctor does not contact you, and a parent has advised you that the student is in treatment, you may choose to contact your fellow professional on your own. In that instance, you would initiate that contact on the understanding that the therapist or doctor may not be able to share any background information with you at all. You may, however, want to let that person know that the student presents certain behaviors or attitudes in your class, and that you would appreciate some additional insight about how you might better serve that youngster in his or her time of need.

At that point, the medical doctor or therapist may choose simply to listen and then offer to get back to you after speaking with the parents. Whether or not you succeed in getting the support you were seeking, you can take comfort in knowing that your own professional observations of the child's behavior may have helped serve the therapeutic goals that had been designed to help the youngster recover and embrace life with all its challenges, rewards, and opportunities.

I have 128 kids, and I see them 43 minutes every day. I have to do lesson plans, correct papers, file mountains of paperwork, go to graduate school, and cope with behavior problems I never even heard of when I was going to school. How am I supposed to find the time to talk to doctors or psychotherapists?

There is no doubt about it: Finding the time to talk to medical doctors or psychotherapists is difficult, no matter what grade or subject you teach. You have to decide for yourself whether the effort ultimately saves or costs you time, effort, and energy. In making that decision, it's helpful to ask yourself some basic questions:

● How much of your time and attention is directed at coping with students who present behaviors that you do not understand and cannot seem to change, no matter what you do?

● Do you prefer dealing with a youngster on the basis of specific information relevant to that student, or do you prefer acting on the basis of what you have learned from general experience?

● How much stress do you experience when your supervisor

asks you to explain why a youngster seems to be presenting behaviors or academic troubles in your class?

● How much anxiety do you feel planning and going through a parent/teacher conference when you can only tell the parent that the child is having trouble, but cannot tell the parent specifically how you plan to help the child do better?

If you feel frustrated because you spend time and attention trying to change behavior or academic achievement and your efforts go unrewarded, then consider how much more gratifying it would be to get some feedback and support from another professional with a different type of insight into the youngster's difficulty. The time you spend would then be productive.

Therefore, you may want to determine how many minutes of every day you spend reacting to or thinking about the youngster's problem. Then take that amount of time and spend it on your own terms, gathering information and seeking support from parents, counselors, supervisors, the child's medical doctor, or the student's psychotherapist. The time you spend actively working to help yourself help the student is an investment that can pay off fairly quickly, since you will begin to cope with that youngster on the basis of information and support, instead of reacting in isolation and without any special insight into the problem.

You may feel that your own professional experience is sufficient to give you the insight you require to help a student succeed in your class. If your education as a teacher included extensive coursework and in-service training in teaching children who present eating disorders, drug involvement, a history of abuse and maltreatment, adolescent adjustment reactions, problems in transition from primary to intermediate level learning, and family difficulties stemming from divorce, death, personal loss, alcoholism, food compulsions, or family violence, then you may be right.

If, however, your training and experience is rooted primarily in the traditional teacher-education curriculum covering the instructional process, human learning, classroom management, child and adolescent development, and curriculum development, plus graduate coursework focusing on children at risk and children with special learning needs, then you may find it useful to try gathering support and information from people who have a different professional background. The burden of teaching children with special needs that interfere with their ability to learn and develop at a healthy pace is so great that the support and information others can provide can be useful and comforting to you.

You may find that support and information particularly valuable when your principal or other supervisor asks you what you are doing to work with a youngster who is underachieving or behaving inappropriately. Remember, your supervisor's training and education is essentially the same as your own. Together, you can approach the child's needs only as you perceive them. If you believe that an additional perspective may give you fresh ideas and support, then seek out the people who can offer you that input. Those people may be school social workers, school psychologists, guidance counselors, special education teachers, administrators, or professionals from outside the school, such as the child's medical doctor or psychotherapist.

If the youngster is not in treatment, you may want to call your local youth bureau, family service agency, self-help group, information clearinghouse, or other public or social service organization to gather some basic information about a problem a student may present, such as sexual acting out, anorexia, bulimia, or drug involvement, to name just a few problems that you may feel a child is experiencing. Remember, your goal would simply be to gather potentially useful ideas and support in your efforts to help the youngster learn and grow. You would not be seeking to diagnose a problem. You would simply be looking for more information than you already have so that you can make an intelligent referral and initiate action. The alternative is waiting to see what the student will do each day and feeling helpless to do anything to assist or stop the youngster.

Your sense of helplessness and lack of information can be a deadly combination in a parent/teacher conference, particularly when the topic is a child's academic or behavioral problems. If you feel helpless and anxious, you may simply feel like telling the parents to get the youngster motivated and organized, to "make" him or her stop daydreaming or calm down in class. Parents may respond by telling you that they do not see that behavior at home, and that may well be true. Or a parent may say, "I'm helpless. I have no idea how to cope with this. I need help!"

Whether you and the parents argue or agree on the issues, you may feel anxious or helpless if you have no new ideas or information to offer those parents. You may find the meeting more productive if you suggest a fact-finding mission, involving yourself and the parents, during which the student, parents, and teacher seek out ideas, feedback, and support from other types of professionals with a different perspective on human development, mental health, physical well-being, or learning.

No matter whether you are in the classroom, the principal's office, a conference with the parents, or a private session with the student, you feel more confident and competent when you know that a student may experience learning and growing problems that simply cannot be helped by a teacher alone. A teacher alone cannot be expected to expend time, energy, and effort trying to resolve issues or problems that he or she is untrained to diagnose or treat.

Do you feel that you spend too much time reacting to demands and needs presented by students, principals, and parents who expect you to know more than you were educated to know? Then learn how to cut down that time by getting support and ideas from the people who are trained to know how to cope with different problems that students may experience in early or later childhood, or in adolescence.

Once you invest your time in gathering support and information from a range of resources, you can start to initiate planned action in the classroom and in those meetings. If you initiate action instead of waiting to see what your student, principal, or student's parents will do, you will have an increased sense of control over your day, and over the integrity of the instructional process as you implement your daily plans. Once you know that you can initiate action and do something to serve the instructional and developmental goals the child must achieve in your class, then you can spend less energy anticipating what problem will crop up next, because you will have acted first. You will have acted on the basis of new ideas and insights from professionals with a different perspective from yours, and you will be stronger for that action.

Because the action you initiate is grounded on information you have gathered regarding how to help that child, you can test the usefulness of the different strategies. As the strategies begin to work, you will expend less and less energy trying to cope with a student's problems, and more and more energy on-task, working with that youngster to help him or her learn and grow appropriately.

The choice is really yours. Spend the time as it is demanded by others, or invest the time according to your own insight and understanding of the students you are responsible for every day of the academic year.

One Day at a Time

Whenever you try a new idea, it's an experiment. It may succeed, fail, or succeed partway. You can protect your own sense of well-being by accepting that reality. If you initiate action to help change something about yourself, your students, or anyone else who is important to you, the whole process is an experiment. It's reasonable to expect that you will have some success if the goal is appropriate and if you understand ahead of time that you may have to adjust the strategies or even the goal itself, in order to achieve that success.

Just keep in mind that change is process. It has built-in ups and downs. Along the way, you may sprint for a distance, and then you may stop. You may have an erratic pace, or you may go along fairly evenly. The fact that you can run one mile in four minutes does not mean that you can run six miles in 24 minutes. You, your students, their parents, and your supervisors share that common human characteristic: We can consider and even act to effect change if three conditions exist:

- We find the change meaningful.
- We understand what the process involves.
- We get the support we need in that process.

You can help support students in their recovery and improvement, if you have the support and information you deserve in order to help that youngster. If no one approaches you with that information and support, then you may find it worth the time and energy to seek it out. You will probably be held responsible for the outcomes, especially if the child fails, becomes ill in your care, or presents chronic behavior problems in class. It's so much more rewarding to be recognized as the person responsible for helping to empower a youngster to learn, grow, and open her eyes to a whole new world of hope.

14 | When You Think Your Friend Has an Eating Disorder

Being a good friend to someone with anorexia is really hard sometimes. It gets confusing when your best friend starts acting as if everything is always just perfect, always smiling and cooking all these elaborate meals, and really showing off how skinny she is. Sometimes I get really jealous of her because she can resist all this food when I'm really hungry...and she stays perfectly thin, like a model. I've seen models like that, and in person, they really look skinny, because the camera adds some weight and makes them look more normal. I know it's dangerous to just not eat, but sometimes it's hard to know what to say or when to say it.

—Marsha Ervin, age 16
Friend of an anorexic girl

If you think your friend is anorexic or bulimic, it's important for you to understand that your friend owns the problem. It is not yours to fix. It will not help if you talk about food and diets forever, or constantly try to make your friends understand that they can die if they continue to play risky games with bingeing

233

and purging. If your friend is sick, you cannot make that person better by continually trying to get him or her to eat the way you think is right. But you can help make your friend see that help is available, and that you will not be part of the problem by talking about food and weight all the time or by admiring dieting that is clearly becoming an obsession. You can become part of the solution by developing your own strategy to cope with the kinds of situations and problems that other people have learned to cope with when they are friends with someone who has anorexia, bulimia, or bulimarexia, or someone who might be at risk of developing such an eating disorder.

When Your Friend Is Starting a Diet

Almost everyone you know has been on a diet, so how can you tell who is or is not at risk of developing anorexia or bulimia? You can't. And you shouldn't try. But you can adjust your attitude toward dieting so that you do not always treat it as a wonderful strategy to improve life.

If your friend says she's starting on a diet, and she is overweight, it would be helpful if you agreed that it was a good idea to go on a diet, but you would like to know more. What are her short-term weight-loss goals? How about the long-term ones? Are they realistic? Has she consulted a doctor? What did the doctor say? What is the doctor's strategy? Is it a really solid one, or is it a combination of too many pills and too little guidance on nutrition and exercise?

What about the diet itself? Is it a balanced combination of diet, sleep, and exercise? Does the diet include a balanced plan for eating protein, carbohydrates, and fats? Or is it a fad diet, promising quick weight loss through fasting, liquid protein, or other tricks that can make the body lose water and muscle first, and fat last?

If you question your friend about the safety and balance of her weight-loss strategy, then you are letting her know that a diet might be a good choice for her physical and mental well-being, if she has a realistic idea of what losing weight will give her. Does she feel that her life will be revolutionized by losing weight? Does she think she will automatically have more friends or better job opportunities because she is thinner? Does she expect people to love her more if there is less of her?

These are danger zones. If your friend expects life and relationships to improve dramatically as soon as she loses weight, then she will probably be angry, bitter, and disappointed when she does achieve her diet goal. Unrealistic expectations for weight loss and life change lead to disappointment, frustration, and cyclical weight gain and weight loss. They can place your friend at risk of developing one or more of any number of eating disorders.

When you question the value of a particular weight-loss strategy, you are also letting your friend know that you care more about her than you care about her becoming fashionably thin. That's a crucial message, because you are refusing to give her permission to lose weight just to gain love or affection. You are giving her permission to lose weight in a sensible way so that she can live a more balanced and comfortable life. But you are also telling her that you care about her just the way she is.

Letting your friend know your concern about the strategy also lets her know that you will not help her fast or shop for foods that represent a completely unbalanced diet. If she says she'll only eat fruit for three weeks until she loses 15 pounds, tell her it's up to her, but you won't be a part of it. You will not admire her for losing the weight, and you will not even acknowledge that she is denying herself other foods she needs and enjoys.

Basically, you will be telling her in no uncertain terms that you care for her too much to allow her to deny herself the right to feel satiated and happy with herself as she loses the weight. Remember, you are not going to tell her whether she's good or bad, or foods are good or bad. All you want her to know is that you care for her, and you will support her in any sensible plan that combines a balanced diet, regular exercise, and sleep. Anything else is unacceptable, because it's dangerous.

Even if your friend ignores your concern and persists in her excessive dieting, you can know that you refused to reinforce behavior that could be dangerous for her. People who develop eating disorders often find permission from friends and relatives who focus so much admiration on the dieting and ability to resist the urge to eat that they forget that the person they care about is literally dying to be thin. If you do not give her permission, and you expect her to be responsible in setting and reaching weight-loss goals, you will not be the one who gives her the permission to possibly destruct.

If your friend tries to draw you into a discussion about food, eating, or dieting, change the subject. Talk about feelings, events, occasions you and she are looking forward to—but avoid getting drawn into a discussion of dieting and food. If she asks which foods are good or bad, discusses food lists, or tries to find out if you approve or disapprove of certain foods, you can advise her that you only know that it's important to eat a balanced diet of carbohydrates, proteins, and some fats, and that a doctor would be her best resource to see if particular foods are or are not good.

You can always include a reference to doctor's care, support groups, and organizations that help people prevent, understand, and overcome anorexia, bulimia, and bulimarexia. Without nagging, you can make it clear that you think it's normal and natural to seek information from every reliable resource before launching on any significant life change, such as a plan to lose weight or eat with abandon without gaining.

Exercise and Eating Disorders

It's nice to exercise with a friend. There's a sense of partnership and competition that can add an edge to the workout and make the whole experience very rewarding, relaxing, and energizing, all at the same time. As with everything else, though, there is such a thing as too much, and there are certain cues that can signal you that your friend's exercise program may not be all that healthy.

Does your friend stay in the sauna for long periods until he sweats off what he thinks is excess water weight? Does she always seem to disappear after she eats a snack or a meal? Is your friend becoming so involved with working out that he seems to be separating himself from his family and his friends outside the gym? Is exercise the only thing that seems to interest her? Does he limit his friendships to those that developed around the gym? Is she reducing the time she needs to spend on school and work so she can accommodate her workout schedule?

If you find yourself answering "yes" to some of these questions, then you may have some cause for concern that your friend's expectations of exercise have gone out of control, with the possible outcome of being part of an eating disorder dynamic. However, it's important to see the danger signs clearly and not imagine that they are present when they are not.

For example, there may be serious cause for concern if your friend is systematically following exercise rituals that exclude family and friends, work and school, and if they appear to be replacing the relationships and activities that used to play an important role in his life. You may also find legitimate cause for concern if your friend keeps upgrading his aerobic workouts in order to keep on losing weight, even though it is absolutely clear that he is too thin and getting thinner.

When an exercise program has a lopsided focus on weight loss and begins to replace valuable relationships and important work or school tasks, then the exercise program is something that you should not approve. If your friend who does not have to lose weight brags continually about how her exercise program helps her keep on shedding the pounds, you do not have to smile or laugh and give your approval. You can ask how all that weight loss and exercise makes her feel.

If your friend keeps on seeking your opinion, you can say

that you are concerned, but that your feelings about his weight and exercise habits do not matter as much as his feelings about himself. By responding that way, you will be helping your friend understand that you are more concerned with him than with his diet and exercise rituals, which are his responsibility. If you clearly demonstrate that you care about him and enjoy his company, but that you believe his diet and exercise behavior is a threat to his health and therefore cannot be admired or discussed at length, your friend will learn that at least one person cares enough about him to concentrate on him, not his bizarre behavior or accomplishments.

If you really do believe that your friend engages in exercise rituals that are not life enhancing, it's important that you do not participate in the same exercises. If, for example, your friend runs ten miles every morning, gets on the rowing machine for an hour in the evening, is about ten pounds below a normal body weight, and still talks about losing weight, you would be giving her your approval if you ran those ten miles with her. When your friend does something self-destructive, it's important to avoid helping her.

That can be a difficult concept to understand, so you might want to consider a different situation. What would you do if your good friend wanted to borrow your car to go to a bar after he had destroyed his own car after driving while intoxicated? If you refused him the car, you would be sending him the message that he was too involved with alcohol to make healthy choices about driving at this point in his life. If you gave him the car, you would be helping him believe that his decision-making skills were good, and that you approved of his previous behavior.

That's how powerful you can be in someone else's life. Your friend can and will interpret your actions as much as he interprets your behavior—if not more so. So think before you participate in behavior that could destroy your friend's health and eventually destroy his or her life.

When Your Friend Is in Therapy

Sometimes, people in therapy talk with their friends about what happens when they go to the doctor or the support group. They may want to find out what their friends think of a particular idea or strategy, or they may be looking for permission either to continue getting healthier or to terminate treatment and remain sick.

If your friend asks what you think about something that happened in therapy, or if she just tells you what is going on, it's important for you to remain nonjudgmental. In therapy, your friend is learning how to make healthy choices based on her own judgment, so you may want to turn the question around— ask her what she thinks. Demonstrate your confidence in her ability to make healthy choices.

Most often, friends do their best job when they help other friends think things through independently. You can raise alternatives, support healthy strategies, or ask if your friend has thought of certain aspects of a problem that she has not yet mentioned. But if you only offer her what you think, she has little opportunity to process your ideas or work on what she really thinks. Then, if she acts on what you think, the outcome of her action will belong more to you than to her. If there is a problem, she can blame you. If she is successful, she can feel that her future success will be dependent on your input. That is an impossible burden for you and a serious deficit for her, since she is the only one who truly has to live with the choices that she makes.

If she complains a lot about her therapist, you can ask her if she has raised these concerns with the therapist. If she says that the group she goes to is not helping her, you can ask her to explore why she feels that way. If she writes from a hospital program and asks you to sneak in food or help her break rules somehow, advise her that you care too much about her to hurt her chances of success in the program. You can also express confidence in her ability to take her complaints and concerns to the appropriate authorities in the hospital, so she can see that you believe she can negotiate for herself when she has a particular need or concern.

Interdependence: The Best of Both Worlds

In friendship, there is no balance sheet. You are generous to each other; you care for each other. But you are two separate people. You cannot make choices for each other, try to control each other, or try to be all things to each other, and still have a healthy relationship based on mutual trust and respect.

Each of you brings something different to the relationship, so it's difficult to decide how much each person contributes to the friendship at any given time. There are times when you will depend on your friend, and times when the situation is reversed. If you find that there is a chronic imbalance in the relationship, then one of you may be substantially dependent on the other all the time, and that is no longer a healthy relationship.

Balance is the central feature of all healthy dynamics, and friendship is no exception. There may be days, months, and even years when a friend requires an extra-special amount of support, and one of those periods could be during treatment. However, you want to be confident that the topics of your conversation, the dynamics of your friendship, and the nature of the balance will change over time, as your friend becomes stronger in therapy.

For example, your friend may be anorexic. When she first goes into treatment, she may focus a great deal of her energy and conversation on trying to get you to play food games. She may want you to join in counting calories and discussing her weight right down to the ounce, just to be absolutely precise about what she does and does not accomplish in therapy.

If she is doing the same things with you six months later, then she may be using you to resist therapy. At that point, you may want to ask her how she feels she is changing in therapy. As she answers you, you can continue to exchange ideas and observations with her, until you have succeeded in expressing your concern about the way the two of you have been interacting. You may both decide to participate in some new activities that will help you break the food-focused rituals that have been characterizing your time together. In doing that, you begin to share new traditions. You show her that you believe the relationship can grow and become more rewarding because the two of you who make up the relationship can grow and feel more rewarded by your own lives, separately and together.

V

PULLING TOGETHER: DEFEATING ANOREXIA NERVOSA AND BULIMIA

15 Pulling Together: Defeating Anorexia Nervosa and Bulimia

Learning to understand and overcome anorexia, bulimia, and bulimarexia is difficult. When these eating disorders affect our families, friends, colleagues, or students, relationships can become strained. Other important issues can be neglected for years while you struggle to cope with a disorder that can compel a person to literally die to be thin.

Newspapers, magazines, and television reports inform us that severe health problems and even death can follow the development of these eating disorders. But most media coverage is limited to news made by people already in the public eye. We developed this book to help you understand that the same eating disorder that destroyed Karen Carpenter can destroy another young man or woman known only to family, friends, teachers, and a handful of doctors.

Anorexia nervosa attacks people who are not rich, famous members of the small class of performing artists. Bulimia can and does destroy the health and lives of people who never make the front page of any newspaper and who may die without anyone's ever really knowing the cause of death.

Just as ordinary people can and do actually die to be thin, they can also lead a life of recovery. Professional help and support groups are available to rich and poor, famous and private. If you are anorexic, bulimic, or both, there is therapy and support that can help you stop starving, bingeing, or purging. If someone you care about appears to be starving, or perhaps engaging in food or exercise rituals that appear to be excessive and highly rigid, you can look for help and find it.

To help make that search less stressful, we have listed resources in the back of this book. If you want to explore even more options, you may get further direction by consulting eating disorders specialists or organizations devoted to helping people understand and overcome anorexia and bulimia.

Sharing information is a step toward prevention, and that is what we have worked to do here. *Share information*. Now you are equipped to share these insights with other people. Maybe you are a teacher in a position of affecting the lives of hundreds of students over the course of your professional career. Find a suitable way to mention this disorder. Whether you are talking about nutrition, health, public affairs, topics for a composition, or weights and measures, you can mention how some people can actually die to be thin, if they do not ask for help.

If you are a parent of a young or older child who you think is already anorexic or bulimic, or at risk of developing such a disorder, you know you can find help. It's as close as the list in the back of this book. Use it. Take advantage of the power you have to affect the situation, even while you understand that you cannot make your child recover. If recovery becomes the subject of a struggle for power, then the recovery is jeopardized. Protect the process. Consult a professional. And if you are not satisfied, keep searching until you find the care that you need. The alternative is to wait for your son or daughter to become progressively worse.

If you are a teacher, then you can be secure in knowing that every time you demonstrate that you believe in a youngster without expecting him or her to be perfect, you participate in prevention. Simply by sending out positive messages about the student's competence and humanity, you have let that child concentrate on success, without hinging everything in life on pleasing you. When you send out a message that every student who does his best has earned the right to pat himself on the back or explore how the success makes him feel, you are telling that youngster that his success is his own—not yours. You are proud, but you want him to do it for himself. That's a message of personal power, and it can translate into positive self-image. A strong, positive view of himself or herself will help your student cope with the strong, negative feelings that every youngster faces in the course of growing up. You have that kind of power.

What if you, the reader, suspect you have one of these disorders? In your heart, you know whether you are becoming ill. You may already know if you have crossed over to a different dimension. You may know if you have put aside relationships, feelings, and physical well-being in order to concentrate all your talent, energy, and creativity on starving, bingeing, or purging. You may know all those things. But now you know that you can change. You know that other people, maybe very like yourself, have faced the same demons and secret voices—and left them behind.

Time matters. The longer you wait, the harder it will be to change yourself. And the harder it will be to empower other people to change themselves. Remember that you cannot change people against their will and expect the change to endure in a positive way. So start with yourself, and find the help you deserve to cope with your own eating disorder, or the difficulties faced by someone you care about very much. Today is a good day to begin.

VI

RESOURCES

ORGANIZATIONS

National and Local Eating Disorders Associations for Referrals, Information, Self-Help, and Newsletters

The four national associations concerned with eating disorders are: Anorexia Nervosa and Related Eating Disorders, Inc. (ANRED); the National Anorexic Aid Society (NAAS); the National Association of Anorexia Nervosa and Associated Disorders (ANAD); and the American Anorexia/Bulimia Association (AA/BA). These nonprofit associations are dedicated to serving individuals and families affected by anorexia or bulimia. In addition, each one of these associations can serve many needs presented by professionals involved in the treatment and prevention of anorexia nervosa and bulimia.

While these four associations provide somewhat different services, most will offer:

- Bibliographies of books and articles
- Printed material about anorexia and bulimia
- Newsletters
- Referrals to therapists and clinics
- Information about public speakers and training programs

It is important for you to understand that each association requires that the therapists and clinics included in the referral list meet high professional standards. However, these associations will offer you the same warning we offer: No one who refers you to a professional person can take responsibility for the treatment outcomes. That responsibility lies with you and the professional person or clinic providing the care.

Naturally, it's also impossible for us to take responsibility for treatment conducted by any program or clinic that we do not work with directly. That is why we strongly encourage you to explore the background and professional standing of the program or private practitioner you choose. That way, you or someone else you care about can be confident that you will benefit from an appropriate treatment plan.

You can reach any of these major information resources by calling or writing the organizations listed below:

AABA CHAPTERS

NEW JERSEY
(NJ only) 800/522-2230
Lisa Citrese, L.C.S.W.
President
AABA of New Jersey
721 Executive Drive
Princeton, NJ 08540
609/252-0202
cbservices@monmouth.com

PHILADELPHIA
Rhoda Kreiner, M.Ed.
Director
AABA of Philadelphia
P.O. Box 68
Wyncote, PA 19095
215/221-1864

LONG ISLAND
Sondra Kronberg, M.S., R.D.,
    C.D.N., President
Eating Disorder Council of LI
82-14 262nd Street
Floral Park, NY 11004
718/962-2778
Web site: *www.edcli.org*

WESTCHESTER COUNTY
Karen Cohen, M.S.W.
Director
Westchester Task Force on
Eating Disorders
3 Mount Joy Avenue
Scarsdale, NY 10583
914/472-3704

NEW YORK REGIONAL GROUPS

ALBANY
Capital Region Association for
  Eating Disorders
79 Central Avenue
Albany, NY 12206
518/464-9043
Info, Referrals, SG

BUFFALO
Eating Disorders Association of
  Western New York
339 Elmwood Avenue
Buffalo, NY 14222
716/885-8834
*Info, Referrals, SG, Free case
management service*

SYRACUSE
Anorexia/Bulimia Support
3049 East Geneseo Street
Syracuse, NY 13224
315/445-1975
Info, Referrals, SG

OTHER NATIONAL EATING DISORDERS ORGANIZATIONS

ANAD
Anorexia Nervosa & Associated
  Disorders
P.O. Box 7
Highland Park, IL 60035
847/831-3438
E-mail: *ANAD20@aol.com*
Info, Referrals, SG

ANRED
Anorexia Nervosa & Related
  Eating Disorders
P.O. Box 5102
Eugene, OR 97405
541/344-1144
Web site: www.anred.html
Info only

EDAP
Eating Disorders Awareness &
  Prevention
603 Stewart Street, Suite 803
Seattle, WA 98101
206/382-3587
members.aol.com/edapinc
*Info, Referrals, SG
Eating Disorders Programs
Associated with Hospitals or
Clinics*

STATE ORGANIZATIONS

PENNSYLVANIA
PENED (PA Educational
  Network for ED)
P.O. Box 16282
Pittsburgh, PA 15242
412/366-9966

COLORADO
Eating Disorder Professionals
  of CO
P.O. Box 18968
Denver, CO 80218
303/649-8561
303/477-0141

MARYLAND
MANNA
(MD Anorexia Nervosa
Association)
410/938-3199

MASSACHUSETTS
MEDA (Mass Eating
Disorders Association)
92 Pearl St.
Newton, MA 02158
617/558-1881

Feeding Ourselves
30 Bartlett Avenue
Arlington, MA 02174
781/643-7977

MICHIGAN
EDEN Club
(Eating Disorders &
Exercise Network Club)
1820 Green Road
Ann Arbor, MI 48105
734/663-4330

MINNESOTA
Alliance to Fight ED
4344 Nicollet Avenue So
Minneapolis, MN 55409
612/824-2353

OREGON
Community Eating
Disorder Treatment Link
503/370-3733

RHODE ISLAND
Anorexia & Bulimia
Association of RI
94 Waterman Street
Providence, RI 02906
401/861-2335

PROFESSIONAL TRAINING & INTERNATIONAL REFERRALS

Academy for Eating Disorders
Attn: Angela Goodus
6728 Old McLean Village Drive
McLean, VA 22101-3906
703/556-9222
E-mail: angela@degnon.org
Web site: acadeatdis.org

International Association of
   Eating Disorders Professionals
123 NW 13th Street, Suite 206
Boca Raton, FL 33432
407/831-7099
800/800-8126

The Renfrew Foundation
475 Spring Lane
Philadelphia, PA 19128
800/736-3739
Training only

CANADIAN ORGANIZATIONS

National Eating Disorders
   Information Centre
200 Elizabeth Street, CW 1-326
Toronto, Ontario
M56 2C4
416/340-4156

Association Quebecoise de
l'Anorexia Mentale et de la
Boulime
8149 rue du Mistral, Bureau 201
Charny, Montreal G6X 1G5
418/832-0574

Eating Disorder Resource Center
of British Columbia
604/631-5313

ANAD
109-2040 West 12 Avenue
Vancouver, British Columbia
V6J 2G2
604/531-2623

PRIVATE RESIDENTIAL PROGRAMS

ARIZONA
Kevin Wandler
Director
Remuda Ranch
Center for Anorexia and
Bulimia, Inc.
10000 North 34th Avenue,
Suite V-400
Phoenix, Arizona 85051
602 861 0600 ext. 4518
1 800 445 1900
remuda@goodnet.com
Web site:
www.remuda-ranch.com

MEDIA WATCHERS

About-Face
P.O. Box 77665
San Francisco, CA 94107
415/436-0212
Web site: *www.about-face.org*

Media Watch
P.O. Box 618
Santa Cruz, CA 95061-0618
831/423-6355
E-mail: *mwatch@cruzio.com*
Web site: *www.mediawatch.com*

Boycott Anorexic Marketing
56 Lothrop Street
Beverly, MA 01915
(contact through MEDA)

Media Education Foundation
26 Center Street
Northampton, MA 01060
413/586-4170

SIZE ACCEPTANCE

Council on Size & Weight
Discrimination
P.O. Box 305
Mount Marion, NY 12456
914/679-1209

Largesse
P.O. Box 9404
New Haven, CT 06534-0404
203/787-1624
Web site: www.fatgirl.com/
fatgirl/largesse/

NAAFTA
National Assoc to Advance Fat
Acceptance
P.O. Box 188620
Sacramento, CA 95818
916/558-6880

The programs listed are just a sampling of those available throughout the United States and Canada. You can find additional information by calling any one of the national associations listed above. Or you could contact your local chapter of the American Psychological Association, American Medical Association, or the National Association of Certified Social Workers. Any one of those sources could provide you with referrals to clinics, individual practitioners, or hospital programs that would be convenient for you.

Remember that this list includes just a few of the resources available throughout the United States and Canada. There are others that may be more convenient or suitable for you, and you can discover where they are located by contacting one of the major national organizations that provide information about:

- Referrals
- Self-help groups
- Speakers with presentations for your group or class
- Newsletters packed with new information
- Support groups for other family members
- Training programs for professionals
- Opportunities to talk with recovering anorexics or bulimics

This list was compiled to help you see how much help there really is for you to understand and overcome anorexia nervosa or bulimia, however it affects you. Wherever you live, you can find support and care from professionals trained to help you or someone you care about who may suffer from anorexia or bulimia. Reaching out begins with just one phone call. It may be the most difficult call you have ever had to make. But it may also be the call that gives you an alternative to dying to be thin.

Books and Other Resources for the General Reader

Chernin, Kim (1981)   *The Obsession: Reflections on the Tyranny of Slenderness* New York: Harper Collins

Coben, Mary Anne   *French Toast for Breakfast: Declaring Peace with Emotional Eating,* New York: The NY Center for Eating Disorders (Published in Spanish as well.)

Costin, Carolyn (1996) — *Your Dieting Daughter: Is She Dying for Attention?* New York: Brunner/Mazel

Davis, Martha et al. [4th ed.] (1995) — *The Relaxation & Stress Reduction Workbook* New Harbinger

Douglas, Susan (1994) — *Where the Girls Are: Growing up Female with the Mass Media* New York: Times Books

Fenwick, Elizabeth and **Amith,** Tony (1996) — *Adolescence: The Survival Guide for Parents and Teenagers* New York: Dorling Kindersley

Freedman, Rita, Ph.D. (1989) — *Body Love: Learning to Like Our Looks & Ourselves* New York: Harper & Row

Goldwasser, Rabbi David (2000) — *Starving to Live*: Judaica Press

Goodman, W. Charisse (1995) — *The Invisible Woman: Confronting Weight Prejudice in America* Carlsbad, CA: Gurze Books

Hall, Lindsey (1993) — *Full Lives: Women Who Have Freed Themselves from Food and Weight Obsession* Carlsbad, CA: Gurze Books

Hall, Lindsey and **Cohn,** Leigh (1992) — *Bulimia: A Guide to Recovery* Carlsbad, CA: Gurze Books

Hall, Lindsey and **Cohn,** Leigh (1991) — *Self-Esteem: Tools for Recovery* Carlsbad, CA: Gurze Books

Hirschman, Jane E., CSW and **Munter,** Carol (1988) — *When Women Stop Hating Their Bodies: Freeing Yourself from Food and Weight Obsession* Reading, MA: Addison Wesley

Hirschman, Jane R. CSW and **Zaphiropoulos,** Lela, CSW (1993) — *Preventing Childhood Eating Problems* Carlsbad, CA: Gurze Books

Holbrook, Thomas, MD — *Making Weight: Men's Conflicts with Food, Weight, Shape and Appearance* (Gurze Books)

Kano, Susan (1985) — *Making Peace with Food: Freeing Yourself from the Diet-Weight Obsession* Boston, MA: Amity

Lauerson, N.H. and **Strukane,** E. (1993) — *You're in Charge: A Teenage Girl's Guide to Sex and Her Body* Fawcett

Lawrence, Barbara Kent (1999) — *Bitter Ice: A memoir of love, food and obsession*: Weisbach Books/Harper Collins

Maine, Margo, Ph.D. (1991) — *Father Hunger: Fathers, Daughters and Food* Carlsbad, CA: Gurze Books

McKay, Matthew, Ph.D. (1994) — *Self-Esteem* Fine Communications

Orbach, Susan (1978) — *Fat is a Feminist Issue* New York: Berkeley Publishing Group

Pipher, Mary (1994) — *Reviving Ophelia: Saving the Selves of Adolescent Girls* New York: Putnam

Rodin, Judith, Ph.D., (1992) — *Body Traps* New York: William Morrow

Roth, Geneen (1982) — *Feeding the Hungry Heart: The Experience of Compulsive Eating* New York: New American Library or Penguin

Ruggles Radcliffe, Rebecca (1996) — *Dance Naked in Your Living Room: Handling Stress and Finding Joy* EASE

Ruggles Radcliffe, Rebecca (1993) — *Enlightened Eating: Understanding and Changing Your Relationship with Food*

Sherman, Roberta Trattner, Ph.D. & **Thompson,** Ron, A, (1997 revised ed.) — *Bulimia: A Guide for Family and Friends* Jossey Bass

Siegel, Michelle, Ph.D., **Brisman,** Judith, Ph.. and **Weinschel,** Margot, Ph.D. (1997 revised ed.) — *Surviving an Eating Disorder: Perspectives and Strategies for Families and Friends* New York: Harper Collins

Schmidt, Ulrike and **Treasure,** Janet (1994) — *Getting Better Bit (E by Bit)* Lawrence Erlbaum Associates

Schmidt, Ulrike (1994) — *Getting Better Bit(e) by Bit(e)* Lawrence Erlbaum Associates

Ward, Susan (1990) — *Beyond Feast or Famine: Daily Affirmations for Compulsive Eaters* Health Communications

Waterhouse, Debra (1997) — *Like Mother, Like Daughter* New York: Hyperion

Way, Karen (1993) — *Anorexia Nervosa and Recovery: A Hunger for Meaning* Haworth

Wolf, Naomi (1992)   *The Beauty Myth: How Images of Beauty are*
[paperback reprint]   *Used Against Women* New York: Doubleday

Magazines

BBW (Big Beautiful Women)

Extra!

Radiance

Videos

Beyond the Looking Glass: Body Image and Self Esteem Hourglass
Productions Inc. 914-723-3065

Body Trust: Undieting Your Way to Health and Happiness narrated by
Gayle Hayes, RD Billings, MT: Body Trust Ltd 406-656-9417

When Food is an Obsession: Overcoming Eating Disorders Hourglass
Productions Inc. 914-723-3065

Women as Large Workout Videos

Slim Hopes: Advertising and the Obsession with Thinness by Jean
Kilbourne Boston: Cambridge Films. 413-586-4170

Professional Booklist and Other Resources

Anderson, A. E. (1990)   **Males with Eating Disorders**
New York: Brunner Mazel.

Belenky, M.F. (1986)   **Women's Ways of Knowing: The**
Development of Self, Voice and Mind
New York: Basic Books.

Berg, F.M. (1977)   **Afraid to Eat: Children and Teens in**
Weight Crisis
Hettinger, ND: Healthy Weight Publishing
Network.

Berg, F.M. (1993)

Health Risks of Weight Loss: 1993 Special Report
Hettinger, ND: Journal of Obesity and Health.

Black, D.H. [Ed.] (1991)

Eating Disorders Among Athletes: Theory, Issues and Research
Reston, VA: American Alliance for Health, Physical Education, Recreation and Dance.

Bloom, C. (1994) et al.
Women's Therapy Centre Institute

Eating Problems: A Feminist Psychoanalytic Treatment Model
New York: Basic Books.

Briere, J. (1992)

Child Abuse Trauma
Newbury Park, CA: Sage.

Brod, H. [Ed.] (1994)

Theorizing Masculinities
Thousand Oaks, CA: Sage.

Brown, C. & Jasper, K (1993)

Consuming Passions
Toronto: Second Story Press.

Brownell, K. & Fairburn, C. (1995)

Eating Disorders and Obesity: A Comprehensive Handbook
New York: Guildford Press.

Bruch, H. (1978)

The Golden Cage: The Enigma of Anorexia Nervosa
New York: Harper Collins.

Brumberg, J.J. (1988)

Fasting Girls: The Emergence of Anorexia Nervosa As A Modern Disease
Cambridge: Harvard University Press.

Brumberg, J.J. (1997)

The Body Project: An Intimate History of American Girls
New York: Vintage.

Chernin, K. (1985)

The Hungry Self: Women, Eating and Identity
New York: Harper Collins.

Chernin, K. (1998)

The Woman Who Gave Birth To Her Mother: Seven Stages of Change in Women's Lives
New York: Penguin Group.

Costin, C. (1997)

Your Dieting Daughter: Is She Dying for Attention?
New York: Brunner/Mazel, Inc.

Courtois, C. (1993) — **Child Sexual Abuse: A Workshop Model**
Milwaukee, WI: Families International, Inc./Family Service America, Inc.

Courtois, C. (January '99) — **Recollections of Sexual Abuse: Treatment Principles and Guidelines**
New York: W. W. Norton.

Emmett, S. (1985) — **Theory and Treatment of AnorexiaNervosa and Bulimia: Biomedical, Sociocultural, and Psychological Perspectives**
New York, NY: Brunner/Mazel, Inc.

Erdman, C. (1996) — **Nothing to Lose**
San Francisco: Harper Collins.

Erdman, C. (1997) — **Live Large**
San Francisco: Harper Collins.

Fairburn, C. & Wilson, G.T. (1993) — **Binge Eating: Nature, Assessment, and Treatment**
New York: Guilford Publications.

Farganis, S. (1994) — **Situating Feminism**
Thousand Oaks, CA: Sage.

Fallon, P., Katzman, M, and Wooley, S.C. (1994) — **Feminist Perspectives on Eating Disorders**
New York: Guilford Publications.

Gabbard, G. & Wilkinson, S. (1994) — **Management of Countertransference with Borderline Patients**
Washington, D.C.: American Psychiatric Press.

Gaesser, G. (1996) — **Big Fat Lies: The Truth About Your Weight and Your Health**
New York: Ballantine Books.

Garner, D. & Garfinkle, P. (1997) — **Handbook of Treatment for Eating** [Eds.] **Disorders (2nd Edition)**
New York: The Guilford Press.

Gilligan, C. (1982) — **In A Different Voice: Psychological Theory and Women's Development**
Cambridge: Harvard University Press.

Goodman, W.C. (1995) — **The Invisible Woman: Confronting Weight Prejudice in America**
Carlsbad, CA: Gurze Books

Gordon, R.A. (1990) — **Anorexia and Bulimia: Anatomy of a Social Epidemic**
Cambridge, MA: Basil Blackwell.

Gottlieb, D. (1991)

Voices in the Family: Healing in the Heart of the Family
New York: Penguin Books.

Harper-Guiffre, H. and MacKenzie, K. R., (1992)

Group Psychotherapy for Eating Disorders
Washington, DC: American Psychiatric Press.

Hatch-Bruch, J. (1996)

Unlocking the Golden Cage: An Intimate Biography of Hilde Bruch
Carlsbad, CA: Gurze Books.

Hayes, D. (1996)

Problems and Exercise Resistance
Lake Dallas, TX: Helm Seminars Publishing.

Hirschman, J. & Munter, C. (1988)

Overcoming Overeating
New York: Ballantine Books.

Hirschman, J. & Minter, C. (1995)

When Women Stop Hating Their Bodies: Freeing Yourself From Food and Weight
New York: Ballantine Books.

Holliman, S.C [Ed.] (1991)

Handbook for Coaches on Eating Disorders and Athletics
Dubuque, IA: Kendall Publishing.

Hornyak, L.M. & Baker, E.K. [Eds.] (1989)

Experiential Therapies for Eating Disorders
New York: Guilford Press.

Hutchinson, M.G. (1985)

Transforming Body Image
Freedom, CA: Crossing Press.

Jacobson, M., Rees, J., Golden, N., and Irwin, C. [Eds.](1997)

Adolescent Nutritional Disorders: Prevention and Treatment
New York: New York Academy of Sciences.

Johnson, C. [Ed.] (1991)

Psychodynamic Treatment of Anorexia Nervosa and Bulimia
New York: Guildford Press.

Johnston, A. (1996)

Eating In The Light of the Moon: How Women Can Let Go of Compulsive Eating Through Metaphor and Storytelling
Secaucus, NJ: Carol Publishing Group.

Jordan, J.V. (1997)

Women's Growth and Diversity
New York: Guilford Publications.

Jordan, J.V., Kaplan, A.G., Miller, J.B., Stiver, I., and Surrey, J.L. (1991)

Women's Growth in Connection
New York: Guilford Press.

Kelly, M. (1996)   **My Body, My Rules**
Planned Parenthood of Tompkins County.

Kaplan, A.S. &   **Medical Issues and Eating Disorders: The**
Garfinkel, P. (1993)   **Interface**
New York: Brunner/Mazel, Inc.

Kratina, K., King, R.,   **Moving Away From Diets: New Ways to**
and Hayes, D. (1996)   **Heal Eating**
Lake Dallas, TX: Helm Seminars.

Lerner, H.G. (1989)   **The Dance of Intimacy**
New York: HarperCollins.

Lerner, H.G. (1998)   **The Mother Dance: How Children Change**
Your Life
New York: HarperCollins

Linden, P. (1995)   **Compute In Comfort: Body Awareness**
Training: A Day to Day Guide to Pain-free
Computing
Originally Published in Upper Saddle River,
NJ: Prentis Hall.
Currently available only from Paul Linden
directly at E-mail Address:
paullinden@aol.com.

Lyons, P. & Burgard, D.   **Great Shape: The First Fitness Guide for**
(1990)   **Large Women**
Palo Alto, CA: Bull Publishing.

Maine, M. (1991)   **Father Hunger: Fathers, Daughters and**
Food
Carlsbad, CA: Gurze Books.

Maine, M. (Summer '99)   **Body Wars: Making Peace With Women's**
Bodies In The New Millennium
Carlsbad, CA: Gurze Books.

Maltz, W. (1992)   **The Sexual Healing Journey: A Guide For**
Survivors of Sexual Abuse
New York: HarperCollins Publishers.

McFarland, B. (1995)   **Brief Therapy and Eating Disorders: A**
Practical Guide to Solution-Focused Work
with Clients
Jossey-Bass.

Pipher, M. (1997)   **Hunger Pains**
Holbrook, MA: Adam's Media Corporation.

Reiff, D.W. &
Reiff, K.K. (1992)

Eating Disorders: Nutrition Therapy in the Recovery Process
Gaithersburg, MD: Aspen Publications.

Rice, J., Hardenbergh, M. and Hornyak, L. (1989)

Experiential Therapies for Eating Disorders
New York: Guildford Press.

Rodin, J. (1992)

Body Traps
New York: William Morrow.

Rubenfeld, I. (1998)

Beginner's Hands: Twenty-five Years of Simple
Somatics: Spring/Summer Issue.

Rubenfeld, I. (1991)

Ushering In a Century of Integration
Somatics: Autumn/Winter Issue.

Ruggles Radcliff, R. (1997)

Dance Naked in Your Living Room: Handling Stress and Finding Joy
Minneapolis, MN: EASE.

Schmidt, U., &
Treasure, J. (1997)

Clinician's Guide to Getting Better Bit(e) by Bit(e): A Survival Kit for Sufferers of Bulimia Nervosa and Binge Eating Disorders
Hove, England UK: Psychology Press/Erbaum (UK) Taylor & Francis.

Schwartz, M.F., &
Cohn, L. (1996)

Sexual Abuse and Eating Disorders: A Clinical Overview
New York: Brunner/Mazel.

Shapiro, F. (1995)

EDMR: Basic Principles, Protocols, and Procedures
New York: Guilford Publications.

Shapiro, F. &
Silk-Forrest, M. (1997)

EDMR: The Breakthrough Therapy for Overcoming Anxiety, Stress, and Trauma
New York: HarperCollins Publishers, Inc.

Siegel, M., Brisman, J. and Weinschel, M. (1997 revised ed.)

Surviving an Eating Disorder: Perspectives and Strategies for Families and Friends
New York: HarperCollins.

Stacey, M. (1994)

Consumed: Why Americans Love, Hate and Fear Food
New York: Simon & Schuster.

Thompson, B.W. (1994) — **A Hunger So Wide and So Deep**
Minneapolis, MN: University of Minnesota Press.

Thompson, J.K. (1996) — **Body Image, Eating Disorders and Obesity: An Integrative Guide for Assessment and Treatment**
American Psychological Association.

Thompson, R.A. & Tratner-Sherman, R. (1993) — **Helping Athletes with Eating Disorders**
Campaign, IL: Human Kinetics.

Times, R. & Connors, P. (1992) — **Embodying Healing: Integrating Bodywork and Psychotherapy in Recovery from Childhood Sexual Abuse**
Safer Society Press.

Treausre, J. (1997) — **Anorexia Nervosa: A Survival Guide for Families, Friends, and Sufferers**
Hove, England UK: Psychology Press/Erlbaum (UK) Taylor & Francis

Vandereycken, W., & Vanderlinden, J. (1997) — **Trauma, Dissociation, and Impulse Dyscontrol in Eating Disorders**
Bristol, PA: Brunner/Mazel, Inc.

Vandereycken, W., Kog, E. and Vanderlinden, M.A. (Eds.) (1989) — **The Family Approach to Eating Disorders**
New York: PMA Publishing Corporation.

Van der Kolk, B. (1996) — **Psychological Training — Co-Editor of Traumatic Stress; The Effect of Overwhelming Experience for Mind, Body, and Society**
New York: Guilford.

Van der Kolk, B., McFarlane, A., and Weisaeth, L. (Eds.) (1996) — **Traumatic Stress: The Effects of Overwhelming Experience on Mind, Body, and Society**
New York: Guilford

Wolf, N. (1992) p/b reprint) — **The Beauty Myth: How Images of Beauty are Used Against Women**
New York: Doubleday.

Zerbe, K.J. (1995) — **Body Betrayed: A Deeper Understanding of Women, Eating Disorders and Treatment**
Washington, DC: American Psychiatric Press.

Zerbe, K.J. (Jan. 1999)   **Women's Mental Health In Primary Care**
Philadelphia, PA: WB Saunders.

Eating Disorders Resources On The Web

Anorexia Nervosa & Associated Disorders (ANAD)
http://www.anad.org/

Eating Disorders Awareness & Prevention (EDAP)
http://www.edap.org/

Anorexia Nervosa & Related Disorders (ANRED)
http://www.anred.com/

International Association of Eating Disorders Professionals (IAEDP)
http://www.iaedp.com.

Academy for Eating Disorders
http://www.acadeatdis.org/

Something Fishy About Eating Disorders
http://www.something-fishy.org/

Massachusetts Eating Disorders Association (MEDA)
http://www.medainc.org/

Eating Disorders Council of Long Island
http://www.edcil.org/

Overeaters Anonymous
http://www.overeatersanonymous.org/

International Eating Disorders Centre
http://www.eatingdisorderscentre.co.uk/

Other Websites

www.aliveness.net

www.open-mind.org

www.empoweredparents.com

INDEX

Binge/purge cycle in bulimia, 4–5, 120
  and anorexia, 24–25
  habit-forming nature of, 1, 5–6, 30
Biofeedback, 155–156, 157–163
Blame. *See* Guilt
Breast changes, and anorexia, 20–21
Bulimarexia, 12, 101–128
Bulimia
  and burst esophagus, 36–37
  compared with alcoholism, 124–125,
    158
  damage done to relationships by, 6
  death from, 162
  defined, 4–5
  development of, 3–4, 5, 118–120,
    158–159
  and dietary supplements, 40
  and diuretics, 32
  early identification of, 33–36
  and electrolyte problems, 39–42, 43
  family reaction to, 121–122
  and heart problems, 39–42
  incidence of, *xiii*
  and laxatives, 32
  and loss of self-control, 120, 122–123
  misdiagnosis of, 208
  and obsession with food, 27
  and parental confrontation, 196–197
  and parnate, 126
  and personality changes, 195–196
  physical dangers of, xiii, 6–7, 33–45
  as "primary disorder," 26
  and secrecy, 5–6
  and search for help, 123–124
  and stress ulcers, 37–39
  and suicide attempts, 161
  and swollen salivary glands, 31, 43
  symptoms of, 194–195
  teachers' testimony on student with,
    207–213
  treatment for, 125–128
  and weight loss, 7, 29–33
  See also Binge/purge cycle; Eating
    disorders; Purging; Testimony, of
    bulimics

Cardiac arrythmia, and eating disorders,
    40, 116
Childhood experiences, and eating
    disorders, *xix–xxi*, 17–20, 144,
    177–182
Clinics, eating disorder programs
    associated with, 251–256
Cold, response to. *See* Thermoregulation
Conflict avoidance
  and eating disorders, 102–105

  marriage relations and, *xxii–xxiv*
Confrontation, 196–197
Constipation, bulimia and, 32
  See also Laxatives
  Cure, recovery and, 184–185

Deaths, from eating disorders, *xii*, 10,
    19–20, 37, 162, 245–246
Dehydration, and diuretic abuse, 32
Dental problems
  and anorexia, 10
  and bulimia, 6–7, 33–36, 39
Dietary supplements. *See* Vitamins
Dieting
  and American attitude toward weight,
    11–12
  assessment of, 97–98, 192
  attitudes toward, 3–4, 233–236
  and development of anorexia, 8,
    53–54, 70–73, 108–114
Diuretics, 32, 196

Eating disorders
  additional reading on, 256
  American culture and, 11–12
  appropriate reaction to, 105–106
  characteristics of, 105–107, 127–128,
    140–142, 193–194
  compared with alcoholism, 105
  and conflict avoiding, 102–104
  and exercise, 236–238
  and fitness obsession, 113–119
  as form or self-punishment, *xx–xxi*
  impact on relationships, 245–247
  increase in, *xiv–xv*
  and motivations for seeking medical
    attention, 133–135
  need for power and, 128
  perfectionism and, 141–142
  postponement of treatment for, 247
  and puberty, 145–156
  reasons for, 14–15
  resources for help with, 249–256
  and role of friends, *see* Friends, role of
  and role of teachers, *see* Teachers,
    role of
  self-destructive impulses and, 128
  treatment of, *see* Treatment of eating
    disorders
  as weapon, 104–105
  See also Anorexia; Bulimia;
    Bulimarexia
Electrolyte disturbances, and heart
    problems in bulimia, 25, 39–43

availability of help for, 246
and difficulties of adolescence, 192–193
and goal setting for children, 191–192
and guilt, 198
role in recovery, 191–201
support groups for, 196–198
teachers and, 208, 211, 217–218
testimony of, 68–100
Parnate, 126
Perfectionism, and eating disorders, 69–70, 106, 126–127, 141–142, 218–219
Permission for dieting, 18, 77, 236
Physical problems, caused by eating disorders, xiii, 6–7, 10, 19–20, 33–45
See also under specific problems, e.g., Dental problems
Potassium, *See* Electrolyte problems
Power, and eating disorders, 128
and attitudes of friends, 238
and biofeedback, 160–161
treatment method and, 140
See also Self-control
Praise, for weight loss, 70–73
Psychologists and psychotherapists and anorexics, 61, 78
biofeedback and, 160–163
teacher's contacts with, 226–227
Puberty
delay in, and anorexia, 20
development of anorexia during, 17–20
and eating disorders, 145–156
parents' problems during, 192–193
Punishment, eating disorders as form of, xx–xxi, 11, 104–105, 126–127
Purging
athletes and, 11, 37–39
and burst esophagus, 36–37
dental effects of, 33–36
and esophagitis, 36
gratification from, 28–29, 118–120, 158
and stress ulcers, 37–38
and weight loss, 29–33
See also Binge/purge cycle; Bulimia

Recovery
parents' role in, 191–201
steps toward, 194–201
teacher's role in, 214
time needed for, 185–187
See also Treatment
Referral, by teachers, 219–223

Relationships, eating disorders and, 6, 110–114, 245–247
Resources for help with eating disorders, 249–256
hospital or clinic programs, 251–256
national and local associations, 249–251
other suggested reading, 256
Rituals, 1, 65, 159
and development of anorexia, 53–54
exercise, 236–238

Salivary glands, in bulimia, 31, 43
School nurse, referral to, 208
School performance, of children with eating disorders, 90–91, 94–95, 208–209
teacher's role and, 223–224
School supervisor, and teacher's role with children with problems, 216, 217, 222–223
Schools, attitude toward anorexia, 94–96
See also School performance; Teachers, role of
Secrecy, of people with eating disorders, xiii–xv, 4, 5–6, 40–41, 58–59, 65
and fear of medical attention, 135–136
See also Manipulative behavior
Self-control
and adolescence, 147–156
and eating disorders, 32–33, 44–45, 91, 120, 122–123, 149–150
and fat people, 50
and recovery, 186
treatment and, 132–139, 159–160
and weight loss in anorexia, 18, 59–60, 75–76
Self-destructive behavior, of people with eating disorders, 128, 159, 236
Self-image
adolescence and, 145–156
creation of, 143–144
eating disorders and, 57, 141–142
and perfectionism, 126–127
Self-love
and eating disorders, xxii–xxvi
and shame and guilt, xviii–xix
See also Self-image
Sexual abuse, 177–182
Skin changes, anorexia and, 7
See also Hypercarotinemia
Sodium. *See* Electrolyte problems
Starvation. *See* Anorexia